"*The Infertility Workbook* addresses a major cause of infertility. It is comprehensive, yet fun and filled with exercises in mind-body medicine that will help you enjoy life even if you aren't trying to get pregnant, and long after you've been pregnant. If you're trying to become pregnant, these exercises will make success more likely. The book also provides useful information on all subjects of concern, including what to look for in Dr. Right."

—Dr. Michael Roizen, coauthor, with Dr. Mehmet Oz, of *You: The Owners Manual, You: Having a Baby,* and *You: Raising Your Child*

"Infertility can take an emotional and physical toll on those couples and individuals who are confronted by a bewildering range of tests and procedures. This comprehensive workbook should be very helpful to anyone suffering from infertility, from the newly diagnosed patient to the IVF veteran. I plan on recommending it to all of my patients."

—John David Gordon, MD, codirector of Dominion Fertility and author of *100 Questions and Answers about Infertility*

"If you are struggling with the weight of the multi-faceted emotional consequences of dealing with infertility, allow Barbara Blitzer's powerful tools to gently yet effectively guide you to heal. Not only will you feel more in control, but you will put the powerful mind-body connection to work to improve your fertility. I encourage you to dive in and get started feeling better now."

—Jennifer Bloome, founder of Anji, Inc., and creator of the *Journey of the Heart* infertility guided-meditation series

"All healing begins within, and the first step toward reproductive health is awareness. *The Infertility Workbook* is an empowering tool that can help women move from a state of fear and deprivation toward one of hope."

—Randine Lewis, PhD, LAc, founder of The Fertile Soul and author of *The Infertility Cure* and *The Way of the Fertile Soul*

"What a relief it would be to have this wise, compassionate, honest, practical guide to navigate the frightening, often disappointing challenges of fertility treatment. This is especially true because Barbara Blitzer writes in her own voice, which feels like having the assistance of a caring, understanding presence, not a distant authority on the subject of fertility. Blitzer's attention to the whole person makes it more likely that couples will come out of this experience gaining personally, whatever the outcome of the fertility effort."

—Ann Ladd, PhD, LCSW, director of The Connecting Place in Pueblo West, CO

"The Infertility Workbook offers a hands-on, down-to-earth practical approach that will inspire those struggling to build their family. Barbara's explanation of the powerful mind-body connection plus the application of her real-world exercises will go a long way toward healing, stress relief, and emotional balance."

—Nancy P. Hemenway, executive director of the InterNational Council on Infertility and creator of the From INCIID the Heart IVF Scholarship Program

"*The Infertility Workbook* is an excellent and essential companion for anyone trying to conceive or experiencing the stress of infertility treatments. It provides a practical, easy-to-use program that can be life-changing. The science behind this mind-body is real and *The Infertility Workbook* offers readers a way to participate in and benefit from sophisticated mind-body programs in the privacy and intimacy of their own homes."

—Elizabeth Swire Falker, author of *The Infertility Survival Handbook* and *The Ultimate Insider's Guide to Adoption*

"I have no hesitation in recommending this book to all who are grappling with the problem of infertility. The book walks the reader through simple emotional and physical exercises that will help establish a healthy mind-body interaction that will assist and empower infertility patients to take charge of their own predicament and render them more responsive to medical treatments. The exercises recommended are well laid-out and easy to implement. I strongly believe that *The Infertility Workbook* will provide a refreshing and much-needed practical contribution to the infertility therapeutic armamentarium."

—Geoffrey Sher MD, executive medical director of The Sher Institutes for Reproductive Medicine and clinical professor of obstetrics and gynecology at the University of Nevada School of Medicine

the infertility workbook

A Mind-Body Program to Enhance Fertility, Reduce Stress, and Maintain Emotional Balance

Barbara Blitzer, LCSW-C, MEd

New Harbinger Publications, Inc.

Distributed in Canada by Raincoast Books

New Harbinger Publications, Inc.
5674 Shattuck Avenue
Oakland, CA 94609
www.newharbinger.com

Printed in the United States of America

Acquired by Jess O'Brien; Cover design by Amy Shoup; Edited by Brady Kahn

Library of Congress Cataloging-in-Publication Data

Blitzer, Barbara, 1945-
The infertility workbook : a mind-body program to enhance fertility, reduce stress, and maintain emotional balance / Barbara Blitzer.
p. cm.
Includes bibliographical references.
ISBN 978-1-60882-009-2 (pbk.) -- ISBN 978-1-60882-010-8 (pdf e-book)
1. Infertility--Psychological aspects. I. Title.
RC889.B57 2011
618.1'78--dc23

2011023270

13 12 11 10 9 8 7 6 5 4 3 2 1 First printing

This book is dedicated to everyone who struggles to have a child, especially all of my wonderful clients, who have trusted me with their stories and made this work possible.

Contents

Foreword vii

Acknowledgments. ix

Introduction 1

1 The Mind-Body Connection 5

2 Understanding Worry 13

3 Seeking Medical Help and Coping With Diagnosis and Treatment 33

4 The Emotional Roller Coaster. 49

5 Connecting to Your Body 75

6 Strengthening Relationships 91

7 Resolution 121

Resources. 133

References 137

Foreword

Stress is ever present in the struggle to overcome infertility. As a practicing reproductive endocrinologist, I have first-hand knowledge of the havoc it can cause in a patient's life.

Multitasking is an art that these patients have mastered. In addition to the demands of their personal and professional lives, they also have to juggle their medical treatments and procedures.

As part of infertility treatment, many patients are referred for counseling and supportive therapies including holistic health procedures such as acupuncture. This workbook is an effective tool to be used by the reader to empower and prepare herself to cope with the demanding infertility experience.

Barbara Blitzer has laid out each chapter in an easy-to-understand format, recognizing that the patient has to lead a normal life despite the demands of the treatment regimens. Understanding the process is important in managing stress and dealing with the anxiety generated by the unknown. The exercises at the end of each section allow the reader to work through several steps in allaying anxiety and taking control of stress.

Recognizing stressors is the first step in any program designed to alleviate stress. This well-researched book helps identify these stressors and then describes individual coping mechanisms.

This book explains in clear language the evaluation and treatment of the frequent causes of infertility. Readers will gain a better understanding of why they have had difficulty becoming pregnant and what options are available to them.

The workbook is interactive and well organized. It offers a sensitive, thoughtful, and pragmatic approach to helping patients become self-reliant and less stressed. It is a book that will provide the reader with "counseling at her fingertips."

I have no doubt that readers will come to rely on this workbook as a valuable resource and use it to nurture themselves as they travel the path ahead.

—Rafat A. Abbasi, MD, FACOG
Columbia Fertility Associates

Acknowledgments

I want to acknowledge my family, who provided support and encouragement throughout this project, and especially my husband, who was most directly affected by late nights and busy weekends. I also want to acknowledge all of those who worked directly on the manuscript, including Herta Feely of Chrysalis Editorial, who assisted at the proposal stage; the wonderful New Harbinger editors, Jess O'Brien and Jess Beebe, who were invaluable during the development stage; and Brady Kahn, my copyeditor. Special thanks go to Nancy Feresten, my brilliant friend who lent her expertise in book publishing at critical moments; to Ann Ladd, friend and mentor, who read the manuscript and offered suggestions; and to Rafat Abbasi, MD, of Columbia Fertility, who provided medical information and support. I would also like to thank my mind-body teachers, Jim Gordon and Mary Lee Esty, and, most of all, Alice Domar for her groundbreaking research on mind-body interventions for fertility.

Introduction

If you're reading this book, chances are you are experiencing anxiety regarding your fertility. You may be, like one in every eight couples, challenged by a period of infertility. You may be worrying about whether you will be able to conceive, even if you have tried for only a short time. You may be worrying about a bleak diagnosis you've just received or about the effectiveness of the treatment you are currently undergoing. Whatever your situation, you are concerned with enhancing your chance of a successful pregnancy. Wherever you are on your journey, this book is for you.

In my many years of working with women and couples, I have found that infertility (or even the worry and anxiety about possible infertility) can become so invasive that it becomes difficult to focus on other things, to maintain a positive outlook, to make plans, or to make decisions. I have also learned that emotional stress or depression can impact outcome. In one Harvard-funded study of women with fertility issues, 55 percent of women who had completed a mind-body program and 54 percent of women who participated in a support group became pregnant within a year, as compared to only 20 percent in a control group that received medical treatment alone (Domar et al. 2000). A more recent study conducted at Boston IVF, a leading fertility center, showed that women who had participated in a stress-management program before or during their second in-vitro fertilization (IVF) cycle had a 160 percent greater pregnancy rate than women who had not (Domar and Nikolovski 2009). A later study of women with no known fertility issues demonstrated that women with increased alpha-amylase—an enzyme marking higher stress levels—in their saliva took longer to conceive (Buck Louis et al. 2010). Other studies have found associations between high stress levels and lower pregnancy rates (Ebbesen et al. 2009).

Although research continues to explore the relationship between fertility and stress, and the answers aren't all in, there are strong indicators that high levels of emotional distress can interfere with fertility and that by taking charge of your emotions, you may improve your chances of becoming pregnant. Simply put, mind-body techniques and emotional support, in combination with healthy, fertility-friendly lifestyle choices, can help you balance your body and your emotions and very likely enhance your fertility.

This book offers you the opportunity to learn and practice mind-body techniques—as I have taught them in mind-body group programs and individual mind-body counseling—systematically, in a way that fits your own situation, without the cost of enrolling in a program, without the structure of a weekly schedule, and without the inconvenience of leaving home. This book will empower you to know yourself and help you alleviate anxiety or depression, whether these feelings are related to infertility directly, tangentially, or not at all. The techniques it offers—including breathing, imagery, working with thoughts, mindfulness, journaling, meditation, connecting with the body, and communicating more effectively—will help to reduce your stress, will make you feel more peaceful and in control, and, even more importantly, may improve your chances of a successful pregnancy.

I have designed this book to be your personal coach, guide, and confidant.

Each chapter provides practical information and anecdotes meant to offer hope and inspiration. The exercises in this book were developed specifically for women with fertility issues, based on my work with countless women experiencing some version of what you are experiencing. Since it is sometimes easier to talk about practicing mind-body techniques than do them regularly, this book will guide you as you learn (and likely struggle) and will encourage you when you are tempted to give up.

My hope is that you will be able to return to these pages over and over again as your journey progresses, repeating exercises and practicing mind-body skills as you need them. Your inner strength and optimism are just like muscles that need to be worked. They will become stronger as you consistently practice them. Furthermore, you will gain a set of skills that will help you not only now while trying to have a baby but also in the future, through whatever life may bring you.

You may have found that your family and friends fail to understand your worries about infertility. They may sometimes say things that leave you feeling hurt and even more alone. You may feel that some of what you are experiencing is either too mundane or too personal to share. The exercises in this book will encourage you to reflect on yourself, your situation, and your feelings. You can respond by writing in the spaces provided, or you may prefer to enter your thoughts in a personal journal. In this sense, the book will be a reliable confidant, and as you reflect on yourself, your situation, and your feelings, it will become a record by which to monitor your progress.

Within each chapter, you will find a Taking Charge section with step-by-step instructions for developing specific mind-body techniques. These techniques are paired with chapter themes but, once learned, can be practiced at any time in your life. This book covers a wide range of fertility topics, and you may want to focus on certain chapters more than others. You should feel free to move flexibly from chapter to chapter, depending on your needs on a given day.

In my own practice, I have seen women struggle with and then be helped by developing mind-body practices. I have seen women move from despair to joy when their dreams came true. At times, I have seen miracles as women who thought they could not conceive went on to have children. At this stage, science does not have all the answers. While I can't predict what fertility outcome you will have, I can promise that practicing mind-body techniques can help you feel calmer, more centered, and clearer.

As one client said after working with me, "I came to you because I wanted to have a baby. Now I have a baby, and I have myself as well." It is my hope that by working in this book, you too will find a more peaceful, skillful self to mother the child who awaits you.

1

the mind-body connection

For many years Western medical practice has separated the mind and the body, underestimating the impact of thought and emotion on physical processes. In recent years, that separation has begun to give way as we have increasingly come to understand the intimate connection between mind and body. Medical practitioners now often recommend counseling and stress reduction to their patients, as integral to good health. This is especially true for conditions, like infertility, in which stress is known to play a role. Whether your fertility concerns are caused by worry, caused by a known medical problem, or unexplained, there is no doubt that infertility is stressful and that you will want to reduce your stress and increase your peace of mind as you try to conceive.

Stress vs. Mind-Body Practice: The Showdown

The relationship between stress and infertility is complex and still under investigation, but when you understand the basics, you can trust that what you are doing to enhance your fertility is worthwhile and has a scientific foundation. Essentially, in order to conceive and carry a baby, you need your hormones to function properly. Estrogen is needed for egg production, and progesterone is needed for implantation of the embryo.

When we feel threatened (or excessively stressed), our bodies naturally react with what's called the *fight-or-flight response*, the exact same physiological response that helped our ancestors escape a charging elephant. When the fight-or-flight response is elicited, everything that's needed for physical survival steps up to the plate. Breathing accelerates, and stress hormones are released to make us fast and strong. The functions not needed for immediate survival are put on the biological back shelf. Digestion shuts down, blood vessels constrict, and the levels of reproductive hormones drop.

The good news is that the practice of mind-body techniques can elicit the opposite of fight-or-flight, called the *relaxation response*, which allows our minds and bodies to rebalance and find a sense of peace and better health (Benson 1983). We now know that meditation and other mind-body practices can even cause changes in our gene patterns (Benson and Proctor 2010). There is also some evidence that these practices can alter the structure and functioning of our brains in ways consistent with reduced stress and greater peace (Seigel 2010; Begley 2007). All of these physical changes help explain the clinical research findings that fertility patients who practiced mind-body techniques were emotionally more balanced, compared with the control groups who had not, even a year after completing a mind-body group (Domar et al. 2000).

In this chapter you will begin to take charge of your stress levels with two techniques that bridge the body and the mind and elicit the relaxation response. These techniques—diaphragmatic breathing and imagery—provide simple but powerful ways to reduce stress.

How Breathing Can Reduce Stress

Breathing usually happens without conscious awareness. You may become aware of your breathing at times if it becomes labored because of physical exertion or is sped up by stressful circumstances, but generally breathing is something that you do without thinking. In fact, the breath is part of the *autonomic nervous system*, which manages blood pressure, the release of hormones, dilation of the pupils, and other internal actions that occur unconsciously.

The autonomic nervous system also controls your responses to stress. It has two branches: the *sympathetic* and the *parasympathetic* systems. The sympathetic nervous system is always on at a low level, but during periods of stress, it kicks into high gear, triggering the fight-or-flight response. The parasympathetic branch is more active when the body is at rest.

Breathing is interesting because it is the one function in the autonomic nervous system that you can control or influence, and by changing the way you breathe for periods of time, you can influence your state of mind. Think of your emotions and your breath as a two-way street. Just as your breathing patterns, speed, and depth of breath will respond automatically to your thoughts and emotions, your thoughts and emotions will respond to your breath if you consciously breathe more deeply. A more relaxed state of mind will equal a more relaxed breathing pattern, and more relaxed breathing will equal a more relaxed state of mind and body. Since the hormonal (or endocrine) system is also part of the autonomic nervous system, it seems logical that by activating the parasympathetic branch of the autonomic nervous system—in other words, by eliciting the relaxation response—you might also influence your hormones. This is one possible explanation for the increased pregnancy rate among participants in mind-body fertility groups.

By working with the breath and with imagery, you can reverse some of the effects of stress on your body. As you practice these techniques in the exercises that follow, notice the changes that you feel. These practices will give your body and your mind a vacation and allow them to relax.

Taking Charge: Diaphragmatic Breathing and Imagery

The way you breathe impacts your emotions, and your emotions impact the way you breathe. When you're stressed, the fight-or-flight response activates and you breathe a very shallow breath that reflects your state of distress and does not oxygenate the lower lobes of the lungs. In true anxiety, you may find it hard to catch your breath, or you may hold your breath to avoid the feeling of anxiety. In a panic attack, people are unable to regulate their breathing and may fear that they're having a heart attack or even that they're dying. Diaphragmatic breathing can reverse these symptoms and bring the body back to a relaxed state.

Breathing diaphragmatically, however, does not come naturally, at least not to adult humans. If you have noticed a baby breathing or even a dog or cat, you may have noticed the belly rising and falling with each inhalation and exhalation. This happens during relaxation when the lungs expand in such a way that the diaphragm descends and causes the stomach to balloon out slightly. Breathing diaphragmatically isn't the way you would tend to breath walking around living your daily life, but as a stress-relieving centering practice, it can't be beat.

Begin your mind-body practice by finding a place where you will be comfortable and where you won't be disturbed. Find a quiet place where you can create a sanctuary of peace.

exercise: Diaphragmatic Breathing

Learning to breathe diaphragmatically isn't difficult. A great way to begin is by simply observing your breath.

Sit or lie down comfortably in your quiet place. Notice where you feel your breath: the nose, the chest, perhaps the back where the lungs are located. Most likely, your breath is somewhat shallow and you are feeling it mainly in the nose and in the chest.

Now rest your hands on your belly. Breathe deeply, allowing the lungs to fill completely. You are directing the breath, but you don't want to stress or strain. Let the breath find an easy rhythm. As you begin to breathe more deeply, you may notice your breath becoming slower as well. Your hands will rise and fall as your belly rises and falls in response to your diaphragm moving down to make room for the lungs to expand. That's all there is to it!

Notice how you're feeling as you breathe deeply. Doing this exercise should make you feel more relaxed as you do it and will also have a relaxing effect on the rest of your day.

When you feel ready to stop, simply return to normal breathing.

Try practicing diaphragmatic breathing daily. You can try it several times a day for short periods. You may want to set an alarm or give yourself another reminder to stop and breathe this way for a few minutes.

You can become more aware of your breath at stressful times and then breathe diaphragmatically to help yourself relax. It's also a good idea to set aside time to practice diaphragmatic breathing in a more formal way. Start with just a few minutes and see if you can work up to ten or, ideally, twenty minutes once or twice a day. Listening to soft music as you do this may help.

Breathing equals being alive. You enter life with your first breath and leave it with your last. If there is anything you already know how to do, it's breathing. Yet, as you have seen by practicing diaphragmatic breathing, you can choose to take an automatically occurring function, the breath, and alter it intentionally to create a desirable result such as relaxation.

Using Imagery to Reduce Stress

Imagery is an automatically occurring process working largely outside of our awareness. Every time you have a memory or you picture a future event, you are creating an image in your mind. You may see it, but you may also sense it in other ways, feeling it, smelling it, hearing it, or even tasting it. Like breathing, imagery can be an amazing tool for relaxation when you take conscious control of it

You may be afraid to try imagery because you believe you're not good at visualizing. Rest assured, you can do imagery whether you're more inclined to visualizing experience, feeling experience, hearing experience, smelling experience, or tasting experience. Imagery includes all of your senses.

Imagery, like breathing, is a great connector. Both breathing and imagery can be thought of as bridges between body, mind, and spirit. Both join the unconscious with the conscious and place important functions under your control. Imagery has often been described as the language of the unconscious. Just as the breath is a two-way street, responding to inner states and also affecting them, the image can express your unconscious and also speak to it. The image can help you change your state of mind and body in ways that other forms of ordinary thought cannot. Imagery is a powerful practice and one that you will surely find beneficial.

The following exercises will help you to elicit the relaxation response while encouraging you to feel safe, strong, and balanced. By simply using this imagery, you can give yourself a minivacation from stress, but without the airfare, days away from the office, interruption of treatment, or disruption of your daily life.

exercise: Safe-Place Imagery

Find a quiet, comfortable place where you won't be disturbed. Focus on your breath, allowing the concerns of the day to recede as you become more and more present in this moment. Take several deep diaphragmatic breaths, allowing each exhalation to be a complete letting go, an invitation to relax and feel the support of your body on the outside, by the chair or sofa or floor, and on the inside by your breath. Experience the pleasure of the breath, the inhalation that nourishes, the exhalation that soothes. Let go. Settle in.

As you become more and more relaxed, more and more at peace, find yourself in a place that is safe and comfortable for you. It may be a place that you've actually visited or seen. It may be a place you've read about, seen in a movie, or even visited in a dream. Your safe place may be on the beach in an exotic place or in your own living room. Where it is doesn't matter as long as you feel safe and comfortable and are in a place where you can be totally at ease. If more than one place presents itself, that's okay. Simply choose one or let one choose you. If you're not finding a safe place, create the one you would like to have. This is your place. You can be alone in it. You can bring anyone or anything into your safe place, and you can remove anyone or anything as well.

Once you're in your safe place, look around. Notice all the sights—the shapes, the colors, the textures, the objects. Take your time looking at all the sights before moving on to notice the sounds, the obvious sounds at first and then the more subtle sounds.

As you are comfortably in your safe place, become aware of the air around you and how it feels as it meets your skin. Is the air warm or cool? Moving or still? Is the air dry or humid? Feel the sensations in your body as it connects with the environment. Feel the sensations of stillness or movement as you then become aware of any aromas in the air and breathe them in, allowing them to deepen your experience of being present in your safe place.

Now, take in your experience of your safe place using all your senses. Allow yourself some time to relax in this place. When you're ready, you can take some deep breaths, stretch, move your body. In your own time, without rushing, you can open your eyes and return to the present moment, bringing with you all that is positive from your experience in your safe place and knowing that your safe place is as close as your breath and your desire to be there.

Reflect on your experience with the safe-place imagery and record your thoughts in the space below.

____

____

____

____

____

Do this exercise often. Your safe place might not always be the same, and that's fine. If at any time you find yourself distressed, you know that you have a safe place to go to. The more you practice this imagery, the easier it will be to create the good feelings each time your return to it.

In addition to feeling safe, you want to feel strong and to build perspective. Imagery can also be empowering. Using your imagination, you can feel as strong as a mountain.

exercise: The Mountain Imagery

Find a quiet place and invite a relaxed state by tuning in to your breath and allowing the body to release its tension. Begin to experience yourself as a mountain, any type of mountain you like. Feel your base as it reaches into the earth. Experience your depth and your solidity as you become aware of your height. Experience yourself reaching deep down into the earth and way up toward the sky even as you become aware of your sides. You may be a mountain covered with trees and other vegetation, or you may be very rocky. Feel your sides, your depth, and your height all at once as you become aware of the season. Notice whether the leaves are on the trees or there is snow on the branches. Perhaps you are so tall that part of you is covered with snow and part of you is enjoying warm sunshine.

Become aware that you have been around a very long time. You have seen the seasons come and the seasons go, over and over again. You hear a bird, you see leaves budding, knowing they will eventually change color and fall. It all changes, season by season. It always has. It always will. See it change, season by season, over and over again. Become aware of yourself. Feel your solidity. You weather it all, feeling your depth, your strength, your height, and your solidity. As a strong and peaceful mountain, you remain.

When you are ready, you can return to the present moment. Take some deep breaths, stretch, move your body, open your eyes.

Reflect on your experience using the mountain imagery. How do you feel after completing it? Draw or record your thoughts in the space below.

____

____

____

____

____

This exercise is another one to practice often. You may find that your mountain imagery will change over time. Your mountains may take different shapes. It doesn't matter if your mountain is round or pointed. What's important is that you find safety and stability inside of yourself.

Experiment with safe-place imagery and mountain imagery, allowing them to transform themselves and to transform you.

Key Points

- The fight-or-flight response occurs with stress.
- Stress affects many physical functions in the autonomic nervous system, including the breath and the endocrine system.
- Stress is thought to change the structure and function of the brain.
- You can counter the stress response by eliciting the relaxation response.
- The breath responds to your state of mind and can also affect it.
- You can use diaphragmatic breathing to create relaxation.
- Imagery is a mental representation of a thought or memory.
- Imagery includes all of your senses, not just the visual.
- You can use imagery to elicit the relaxation response and create a positive state of mind.

2

understanding worry

If you've begun trying to conceive and it's not happening as you'd hoped, worry is natural and legitimate. Ever since you were a little child, you have assumed that one day you could choose to be a mother. You may have played with dolls, thinking that one day you would have real babies. It's likely that you're now thinking of pregnancy after having achieved other important goals. Perhaps you've found the partner you were looking for, the one with whom you would like to start a family. Perhaps you have achieved professionally and now feel you can make time and space for a child. You may have simply reached an age and time when you feel ready to be a parent.

Whatever your specific circumstances, if you want a child and aren't sure you can conceive, you are, of course, going to worry. You may feel that having a child is the first important life goal that you can't achieve through hard work. You may feel that you've lost control of a central part of your life. The combination of your strong desire and the uncertainty of the outcome sets the stage for worry. It's the perfect worry equation: high vulnerability plus low control equals worry (Hallowell 1998).

But even though it's natural to worry when dealing with infertility, no one can say it's pleasant. This chapter can help you learn about yourself and develop skills that can reduce your worrying. By exploring the specific content of your worries, as well as any mental or emotional tendencies that might be contributing to worry, you can gain greater understanding and, with it, greater emotional control. As you face your fears and evaluate the evidence for your worries, you will be able to decide how much weight to give them. Knowing the difference between your fears and the facts will help you be in the present—rather than in a projected future that may never occur—and enable you to develop more effective coping strategies.

This chapter begins with an outline of the worries that many women encounter when having fertility challenges. In the exercises that follow, you can explore which of these worries resemble your own and whether you have a tendency to worry that may be informing how you are feeling. The more you know about yourself and how your mind operates, the more in control you will feel.

The Taking Charge section in this chapter presents two very different strategies for conquering worry. The first is to use *cognitive behavioral therapy* (CBT)—which works with your thoughts to improve your mood—to help you address and evaluate your worries directly. The second is to employ mindfulness to move away from worries about the future into a fuller, more peaceful experience of the present moment. These two strategies complement each other, and using both can have a very powerful effect.

Common Worries

The worries mentioned here are the ones I hear most from women with fertility concerns, and some of them probably reflect your worries. So know that you are not alone. Others who face what you are facing have had the same worries, and most have come out on the other side. Noticing your reactions as you read the paragraphs below and then completing the exercises will help you know more about what you are dealing with.

You also may discover that you have some worries that are all your own. That's okay. No matter what's worrying you, you can use the techniques that are offered here to get the better of your worries.

Worrying about Being Left Behind

The fear of being left behind is a common one. You may feel like you've been left on the platform while others are on the train heading off into a future you hope for but which may seem uncertain. It may seem that there's a mom's club that you can't get into. Your social life may change as your friends' interests and conversations are increasingly about babies and children. If many of your friends have children, they may be less available to you because they're busy with child-centered activities, or you may find that spending time with them is less rewarding—or even painful—for you.

If this is happening in your life, you may be feeling alone and worried that it won't change. You may be concerned that even if you do get pregnant, your children won't be the same age as those of your friends or siblings. If you do have siblings, especially younger siblings, who are getting more visits and more attention from your parents in their new role as grandparents, you may worry that you have become less important in your parents' lives. Watching your friends and perhaps family members getting pregnant can be excruciating.

Worrying about Self-Worth

If you're worried about fertility, you may also worry about your personal adequacy. Although fertility problems are common and don't reduce your value as a person in any way, your self-esteem may nonetheless suffer. You may feel that your body has betrayed you or believe, incorrectly, that you are less of a woman because your body isn't performing as you would like. You may fear that you will be unable to ever experience pregnancy and childbirth. Self-blame is common among women who fear that they waited too long to try for a baby and especially among women who have had earlier abortions. Some women believe they are being punished for something they thought or did earlier in their lives. If you're very worried, you may feel that your personality has changed and that you're less fun to be with, which can create even more issues with your sense of who you are as a person.

Worrying That Your Relationship Will Change

Regardless of who you think has the fertility issue—you, your partner, or both of you—tensions and fears may develop in your relationship. Your lovemaking may change as sex becomes more goal directed. Many women and men complain about having to have sex for baby making and that sex at other times tends to remind them of their fertility problems.

Feelings in your body as a result of fertility treatments, as well as emotional responses to infertility, might dampen your personal relationship. If you feel that your body has betrayed you and are worried that you might not experience pregnancy and childbirth, it may be more difficult to enjoy your body.

If the fertility problem is identified on your side, you may feel broken or not as feminine as you once did. If it's on your partner's side, you will have difficult feelings to reckon with as well. Unexplained infertility can be frustrating too because you may wonder if you have a problem as a couple. Sharing common worries may bring you closer together, but it may also make communication difficult and create stress.

Worrying about the Future

Besides being uncomfortable in your current life, you may project your worries far into the future. You may worry about a childless future, or if you're thinking of other options, such as adoption, donor egg or sperm, or surrogacy, you may worry about the implications of those possibilities. Many of my clients couldn't imagine any happiness in their lives without biological children. They look way off into the distance and create sad scenarios for every stage of life. You may also be worried about being middle-aged with no children, old with no grandchildren.

While these worries are normal and understandable, there is an excellent chance that the scenarios you torture yourself with will never come to pass. If you're so preoccupied with worries about fertility and its possible impact on your future, you can't concentrate or enjoy your life in the present.

The following exercise will help you determine which, if any, of the common worries mentioned in this chapter apply to you.

exercise: Name Your Worries

Take the following steps to name your worries and reflect on your feelings:

Review the worries outlined in this chapter. Now, consider your own life, your own friends and family. In the space below, list your worries specifically. Name your fears. Be as clear as possible. Name people in your life if doing so seems applicable. For example, do you have siblings with babies, and does this make you feel left behind? If so, who are they and how do you feel about them? Or has anything changed in your social life? With whom? What's happening at work? Any baby showers? Are you worried about yourself or your relationship? Take your time and write about what's happening in your life or what you fear may happen. Remember, this is just a starting point, and there will be many exercises in this book to help you work through these issues.

____

____

____

____

____

Ask yourself if your worries are more about what is happening in your life at present—such as dealing with pregnant friends—or if they are more about what you fear for the future. As you review your list, mark your worries with either an N for now or an F for the future. How far into the future do you imagine your life?

____

____

____

Although the future may be uncertain, you do know that whatever you are currently experiencing will change. This is a time in your life that you are passing through, not your whole life. There will be a resolution. In the meantime, are you experiencing all that is good and beautiful in the moment, just as it is, or are you living an unhappy future that may never be?

Do You Have a Worry Habit?

If you're a worrier in general and now have a fertility concern, you may be suffering more than necessary. The fact that you are very worried about having a baby doesn't actually prove that it will be difficult for you to have a baby. You may be worrying a lot and still have a good chance of becoming pregnant.

Some women with fertility issues have been trying to conceive for a long time without success but remain relatively calm and optimistic about their futures, while others panic after what may be only a minor setback. If you're a worrier by nature, you most likely have mental and emotional habits that are not serving you well at this time. Sometimes a worry is well founded and predicts an event that must be accepted, but if you have a worry habit, as many people do, you may find that much of what you worry about never comes to pass. You may be like Beth.

Beth's Story

Beth was breathless when she first called my office for an appointment for infertility counseling. She tearfully explained that she had had menstrual irregularities in the past and now had been off birth control and trying to get pregnant for three months. Her younger sister had just announced that she was pregnant, and her parents were totally focused on the prospect of becoming first-time grandparents. Beth was convinced that after three months of frustration, she was headed for infertility and would have to have the infertility treatments that she feared. She was having difficulty sleeping and found it hard to concentrate at work. Many of her friends had babies, and she was avoiding them. She realized she hadn't tried for that long, but she said that she had a sense of doom about her prospects. Having a baby was something she had always really wanted, and she was very afraid of being disappointed.

In counseling, Beth talked through her issues. Telling her story helped her release tension and feel less alone. Cognitive behavioral approaches gave her the tools she needed to evaluate her fears in terms of the facts and to reframe her thinking. Beth had been repeatedly rehearsing the future that she feared. To counter this tendency, she also learned some relaxation and mindfulness techniques to help her experience and accept the current reality of her life, which was happy overall.

After three more counseling sessions, Beth called to say that she was pregnant. She continued therapy well into her pregnancy, which brought its own worries and concerns. As Beth successfully incorporated a mind-body program into her life, her overall tendency to worry diminished. She was far more able to think realistically, to live mindfully in the moment, and to anticipate her future with pleasure and confidence. I like to imagine her now as a mother, sharing her clear thinking and calm confidence with her new family.

exercise: Are You a Worrier?

Take the following steps to determine if you tend to worry:

1. In the space below, make a list of things you have worried about in the past. For example, you may have worried about finding a spouse, the right job, a house you liked. If you're the kind of person who tends to worry a lot, you may be able to find small events that caused you intense distress.

   ____

   ____

   ____

2. For each worry, try to recall the event in detail and rate the intensity of your distress on a scale of 1 to 10, where 1 represents the smallest amount of distress and 10 the greatest.

   ____

   ____

   ____

3. Finally, note whether or not the thing you worried about ever happened or if it happened in the way you feared.

   ____

   ____

   ____

Review this list of worries and think about whether or not you are someone who generally worries a lot. Do your worries overall tend to predict a future event accurately, or do your worries more often turn out to be just worries?

Most of us worry about things that never happen. The women I've worked with over the years have worried that they would never have happy families, and yet I could paper a wall with the photos of babies these women later mothered. The future is unknown, of course, but if you see that you have worried about a lot of things in the past that never occurred, it may comfort you to know that your emotional reaction right now may be another expression of your tendency to worry and not an indicator of what your fertility outcome will be.

If you are a worrier, the next exercise will help you be more realistic about the relationship between your worry and what you know about your fertility. Later in this chapter, you will have a chance to do more exercises to combat your worrying.

exercise: Write a Letter to a Friend

In the space below, write a letter to a loving and compassionate friend—this friend can be imaginary—telling the story of your life in relationship to worry. Do your worries overall tend to predict a future event accurately, or do your worries more often turn out to be just worries? Do you remember worrying as a child? Do others in your family worry a lot? Did anyone ever comment on how much you worry? Has anyone ever described you as calm and easygoing? Would you describe yourself as generally optimistic or pessimistic?

Now switch places and pretend that you are the loving and compassionate friend who will receive this letter. How would you respond? What would you say to your friend who tends to worry?

If you believe that you worry more than you would like, be as compassionate and gentle with yourself as you would be with a dear friend.

If you are a worrier, remembering Beth's happy outcome may help calm your fears. You may be able to say, "I know I worry a lot. Many of the things that I've worried about happening in the past have never happened. Maybe the things I fear now will never come to pass. Let me gather some more information and see what the future brings."

When Worry Is Extreme

It's important to be able distinguish worry from depression. Worry can be defined as concern about an issue that has an uncertain outcome. Mild worry is normal and not harmful. When worry and stress become extreme, however, they can lead to *clinical depression*, a medical condition that threatens your ability to function effectively in several areas of life. It's emotionally painful and has physical symptoms.

There are two types of clinical depression. *Major depression* is a debilitating condition that threatens the depressed person's ability to live effectively. Major depression can appear suddenly and be quite dramatic. *Dysthymia* is a less extreme form of depression but one that is unpleasant and long lasting. In fact, to be diagnosed with dysthymia, you must have had symptoms most of the time for at least two years. The following exercise may help you determine if you are suffering from some of the symptoms of depression.

exercise: Are You Depressed?

Answer the following questions yes or no:

1. Do you feel sad most days of the week? Do others think you seem down most of the time?
2. Have you lost interest in the activities that used to bring you pleasure?
3. Have you gained or lost weight recently without trying to? (Here, don't count any weight changes that might have occurred as a result of fertility treatment. This question refers to changes in weight that may be related to eating or loss of appetite due to emotional issues.)
4. Do you have trouble falling asleep or staying asleep? Do you want to sleep much more of the time than you did in the past? Do you have trouble falling asleep or staying asleep most days of the week?
5. Do you feel agitated and need to move your body a lot?

6. Does your body feel heavy and lethargic, making it difficult to move around and do things?
7. Do you feel fatigued or lack energy most days of the week?
8. Is it difficult to think, concentrate, or make decisions most of the time?
9. Do you feel worthless or guilty much of the time?
10. Do you feel hopeless or have thoughts of death or suicide?

This list of questions reflects the symptoms of major depression (American Psychiatric Association 2000). If you answered yes to two or more of the questions, I urge you to see a mental health professional to determine whether you may be suffering from some form of depression.

While it is common for women experiencing infertility to feel stressed and even somewhat depressed, if you think you may be clinically depressed, it is important to seek help. In addition to making you feel bad, depression can create changes in your body that may not be conducive to fertility or your overall health.

There are many therapists who focus on fertility issues. Through your local chapter of Resolve (and infertility information organization) or through the American Society for Reproductive Medicine (ASRM), you can find therapists who have special expertise in working with fertility issues (see resources). Your doctor may also be able to refer you to a therapist. You may also want to consider joining a support group in your community; even an online outlet for your feelings can be relieving and helpful. It's important to have people who understand what you're going through. There's no need to go it alone.

If you're considering taking—or you are already on—medication for depression, and you're trying to conceive, you should consult with your doctor about the best course of action. Although I use mind-body approaches to help my clients alleviate depression, there are certainly people who benefit from a combination of medication and mind-body approaches, and I encourage my clients to discuss all options with their doctors. There are antidepressants that are considered safe during pregnancy, but a decision to use them is very personal.

The good news is that whether or not you decide to seek additional help for depression, there is evidence to suggest that mind-body exercises can help. In one study, the women most depressed at the beginning of a mind-body group conceived at the highest rates after completing the group (Domar 2002). The researcher's assumption was that reducing depression through the mind-body program created the dramatic increase in fertility. Alleviating depression is an important part of your mind-body fertility program and may improve your fertility as well as your mood.

Taking Charge: Cognitive Behavioral Therapy and Mindfulness

Two very different but complementary mind-body approaches can help you reduce your worrying and the stress that accompanies it. A cognitive behavioral approach can help you distinguish worry from fact through an evaluation of your thought processes. This approach can help you develop realistic optimism while dealing with the uncertainties of infertility. Next, you can use mindfulness to move away from worrying about future events that may never occur and toward a fuller experience and acceptance of the present moment. Some things can't be changed, but our way of experiencing them often can.

Reducing Worry with Cognitive Behavioral Therapy

Cognitive behavioral therapy can help you look at your situation, whatever it may be, with more objective eyes. CBT asks you to evaluate your thought processes and to look closely at how you arrive at your conclusions. Some of your conclusions may be realistic, but others may come from thinking in ways that are neither helpful nor accurate.

When you're stressed out from dealing with infertility, you may not be aware that you're more susceptible to distorted, scared thinking. But if your thinking is affected by stress and worry, CBT can help you pull in the emotional reins and think more clearly. You'll find it to be a great tool now and in the future.

Cognitive behavioral therapy is based on the understanding that what we think has a lot to do with how we feel and that our thinking isn't always accurate. CBT has been demonstrated to be an effective treatment for both depression (Dobson 1989; Hollon et al. 2005) and anxiety (Gould et al. 1997; DeRubeis and Crits-Christoph 1998; Durham et al. 2003; Borkovec and Costello 1993). One of the best things about CBT is that it offers a step-by-step process for examining your thoughts and working with them in ways that improve your mood while encouraging you to be realistic. The first step is to identify your worry thoughts. (You already began to do this earlier in this chapter.) The next step is to look at whether your worries represent certain mental habits or thought patterns that may be causing you trouble. The third step is to examine the evidence for and against your fears. The fourth step is to generate more positive ways of looking at the situation. The final step is to reframe and restructure your thoughts to be more positive without being unrealistic about the challenges that lie ahead.

Looking at Mental Habits That Can Cause Trouble

The following thought patterns are known in CBT as *cognitive distortions*, which are unrealistic yet repetitive ways of thinking that can have a powerful influence on your mood. As you read about these thought patterns, see if any strike you as your frequent default mode of thinking when under stress. If the examples given below seem too extreme to you, and you find yourself saying, "I don't think this way," consider whether you might use some of these thought patterns in more subtle ways or in different situations. Remember, it's great if you can identify unhelpful ways of thinking, because doing so will lead to some answers for how to lower your stress.

All-or-nothing thinking. All-or-nothing thinking means seeing the world in black-and-white extremes. Things are either all good or all bad. All-or-nothing thinking often seems like fact when it isn't. Thoughts like "my life will be over without a child" or "I can never be happy without a biological baby" are unrealistic for most people, although they often feel like absolute fact. Most people are able to move through an infertility crisis and find resolution one way or another.

Overgeneralization. Overgeneralization occurs when you decide that something always or never happens because it has or hasn't happened in some instances. For example, if you've had a very long wait at your doctor's office for two out of six visits and conclude that you always have to wait forever, you are overgeneralizing. If your partner doesn't understand your feelings on a particular topic and you conclude that he never understands you or always misunderstands you, you are also overgeneralizing.

Mental filtering. Mental filtering means blotting out positive information to focus exclusively on the negative. If, after an unsuccessful in vitro fertilization, your doctor tells you that he or she has a new protocol that might be effective for you, and you come away thinking only that in vitro fertilization doesn't work for you, you are engaging in mental filtering. You are thinking about what didn't work and not hearing the possibilities that have opened as a result of the new procedure.

Discounting the positive. Discounting the positive means minimizing what is good and emphasizing the negative. You haven't totally filtered the positive out of your awareness, but you don't give it adequate weight. If, in the previous IVF example, you hear that there is a possibility of a new protocol but give that fact very little weight, you are discounting the positive.

Overestimating the threat. You may be overestimating the threat if you take information that implies a slight risk and magnify that risk into something terrible and frightening. For example, if one of your friends became emotional after taking fertility medications and, as a result, you decide you will suffer major depression as soon as you enter treatment, you are most likely overestimating the threat.

Catastrophic thinking. In catastrophic thinking, you take minor setbacks or difficulties and from them imagine horrible or unbearable outcomes. Perhaps you've been trying to conceive but with no success and you're frustrated and scared. If you then were to decide that you will never be a mother and that your life will always be totally miserable, you would be engaging in catastrophic thinking. If words like "horrible," "terrible," and "ruined" have become common in your thoughts, this is a clue that your thinking is catastrophic in tone.

Fortune telling. Fortune telling means predicting the future and believing you must be right. Fortune telling may be one of your favorites as you deal with fertility, and you may predict the future in negative terms although that future is still unknown. But with infertility, only uncertainty is certain. If you're working in this book, you most likely don't know what your future family will look like or how it will be built.

Should-statements. You may notice that you're falling into this thought pattern if you hear yourself talking to yourself about how you should feel and what you should do. For example, if you think that you should go to all your office baby showers and should not feel envious, you are being constrained by rigid ideas that aren't helpful.

What-if thinking. In this sort of thinking, you scare yourself by imagining negative future scenarios. What if I never get pregnant? What if my husband leaves me because I can't get pregnant? What if I use up all my money on fertility treatments, and we don't buy a house now, and the economy gets worse, and I can't afford treatments, and I turn forty and my fertility drops, and I'm the only woman without a child and the only person without grandchildren, and I'm all alone in a rented apartment in my old age? What if? One of the problems with what-ifs is that they can snowball into catastrophic thinking and leave you feeling really bad about events that will probably never occur.

Discounting coping resources. You may underestimate your ability to handle challenges effectively. Okay, what if you don't get pregnant? What if you don't get exactly what you want? Do you think you can build a family another way? Do you think you could grieve the loss and find a satisfying life? Or do you see yourself as devastated for life? Most people have more ability to cope with disappointment than they realize.

Examining the Evidence

Once you have identified your worry thoughts and worry-thought patterns, you can begin to question the evidence for and against your fears. For example, if you fear that you'll be left behind by all your friends who are having babies, you would think about your friends as individuals and notice that each friendship is unique. You could evaluate which friends have been with you through other life changes, such as finishing school, getting a job, or marrying, and ask yourself how likely it is that you or they would want to end the friendship based on your family status. If you have seen certain friends less often while dealing with fertility issues, you would ask yourself why that is and whether you think it's something that will continue in the future, once your fertility issues are resolved.

Generating More Positive Ways to Look at the Situation

The next step is to think of other possibilities. Again, say your fear has been that you're going to lose all your friends. In this step, you would decide which friends you want to be around and what you have in common apart from whether or not you have children. You might remind yourself that your situation is temporary and also that you have a lot of control over which friendships continue.

Reframing Your Thinking

The final step is to create a new thought. Instead of thinking, "I'm going to lose all of my friends," you might reframe your thinking as follows: "Some of my friendships may change for a while or even permanently, but the friendships that are important will remain. I have a lot of control over developing and maintaining friendships, whether old or new. Right now, I'm focused on fertility and am worried about how I will build a family, but in the future, the issue will be resolved, and most likely I'll have children of my own and be comfortable with my friends."

exercise: Reframing Your Thinking

As a cognitive behavioral exercise, take the following steps to reframe your worried thinking habits about infertility:

1. Identify your worried thought. Name a worry that you have related to infertility, such as "I'm afraid I will never become pregnant, and ______________________________________." Fill in the blank with what you worry about.
2. Look for and name any cognitive distortions in your thinking. Use the preceding list of cognitive distortions as a guide.
3. Ask yourself what evidence exists for your fears. Give evidence for and against your worried thought.
4. Try to generate more positive ways of looking at the situation.
5. Write your reframed, hopefully happier, thought. Actively try to substitute this thought for your worried thought if the worried thought reappears.

Use the following space to practice reframing your own worried thoughts. Identify your top three fertility fears and then work with one worried thought at a time.

Your worried thought: ____

Cognitive distortions: ____

Evidence for and against ____

Other possibilities ____

Your reframed thought: ____

Your worried thought: ____

Cognitive distortions: ____

Evidence for and against ____

Other possibilities ____

Your reframed thought: ____

Your worried thought: ____

Cognitive distortions: ____

Evidence for and against ____

Other possibilities ____

Your reframed thought: ____

The following story shows how one client was able to use cognitive behavioral therapy to address her cognitive distortions and reframe her worried thoughts.

Erin's Story

When a therapy client named Erin did this cognitive behavioral exercise, she listed her top three worries as follows:

1. *"I'll never get pregnant."*
2. *"If I don't have a baby, I'll never be happy."*
3. *"Infertility treatments can't help me. I'll be the only woman I know who wants to be a mother and doesn't succeed."*

Erin then reviewed her three fears and identified the cognitive distortions that were behind each fear.

1. *"I'll never get pregnant.": fortune telling, overgeneralization, catastrophic thinking*
2. *"If I don't have a baby, I'll never be happy.": catastrophic thinking, fortune telling, overgeneralization, minimizing coping skills*
3. *"Infertility treatments can't help me. I'll be the only woman I know who wants to be a mother and doesn't succeed.": fortune telling, overgeneralization, catastrophic thinking*

The fears and cognitive distortions that Erin was facing are common ones and might well be yours. These worries cause real pain, and they represent possibilities feared by most of the women I've met with. The problem is that for women who lean toward worry, fears about possibilities can begin to seem like fact.

After listing her fears and identifying her cognitive distortions, Erin looked for evidence for and against her fears, generated more positive ways of looking at her situation, and reframed her thoughts to have a more realistic and positive outlook. Here's what Erin came up with:

Worry: *"I'll never get pregnant."*

Evidence for and against: *"I may never get pregnant, but there's a good chance that I will. If it were hopeless, I wouldn't be starting a new IVF cycle. There is no evidence that I won't get pregnant. In fact, my doctor is giving me a 60 percent chance, so it would be more realistic for me to say I will get pregnant than I will never get pregnant."*

Other possibilities: *"If my next IVF isn't successful, it's possible there will be a new protocol we can try. But then again, it may work. The truth is, I don't know what will happen in the future."*

Reframed thought: *"I have a good chance of getting pregnant. I'm doing everything I can to make it happen. Many women have gotten pregnant after a few failed cycles."*

Worry: *"If I don't have a baby, I'll never be happy."*

Evidence for and against: *"There is no evidence that I won't be happy in the future. I actually don't know how I'll feel. I'm projecting my feelings now into the future."*

Other possibilities: *"I've heard that many women in this situation later become happy in ways they never imagined they could be. Yes, when they think about it, they are disappointed they didn't have a 100 percent biological baby. Some have had babies with donor eggs or donor sperm or through adoption and are very happy. Now that they're here, they love their children and their lives. Others have decided to accept that they won't have children and are having rich, full lives, traveling with their spouses, childfree. There are many possibilities for happiness. If it doesn't happen in the way I hope, I have other alternatives for building my family. I can learn to be happy with other options because I have known myself to have good coping skills in many situations. I will be very disappointed if I can't become pregnant, but I will be able to cope. I know I will love any future child I have and I can make a good life for myself and my family, with or without children."*

Reframed thought: *"I hope to have a 100 percent biological child and am doing all I can to make that happen. Even though I know I'll be disappointed if I have to find an alternative way to build my family, I know I will adjust and find happiness. In the meantime, I remain optimistic."*

Worry: *"Infertility treatments can't help me. I'll be the only woman I know who wants to be a mother and doesn't succeed."*

Evidence for and against: *"There is no evidence that my doctors can't help. Just because I've had a couple of failed cycles doesn't mean I won't succeed."*

Other possibilities: *"Many women have had success after a couple of failed cycles. I've even been told that we're trying a new protocol next time, which should increase my chances. Also, I'm working with mind-body techniques and, overall, I feel less stressed. I know my doctor would not be working with me if I didn't stand a good chance of success."*

Reframed thought: *"I'm in the process of trying to conceive with the assistance of an excellent team of doctors who think I have a good chance of success. I'm increasing my statistical odds of success by practicing mind-body techniques and have reduced my stress."*

When dealing with fertility problems, there are many unknowns. The key is to minimize any tendency to predict a negative future when you in fact don't know what your outcome will be. When you think a worried thought about the future, ask yourself what the evidence is for and against that outcome, try to look at other possibilities, and if your worried thought has been causing you stress, encourage yourself to reframe it and let it go.

Meeting Worry with Mindfulness

Mindfulness as used in this book applies to the formal and informal practices derived from Buddhist practice, as well as to other mind-body practices such as yoga, imagery, and relaxation. There are many styles and schools of meditation and stress reduction, but they all have overlapping components. Experimentation and practice will bring you to a personal knowledge of what is most helpful to you. Whatever you are doing, being in the moment—being present—is key.

Mindfulness is the perfect antidote to worry (Kabat-Zinn et al. 1992). Over time, it will help you find a calm center. Mindfulness is a way of living in the world and being present to what is. While worry takes us into an unknown future that we embroider with our fears, mindfulness is about being firmly in the present without filter or judgment or striving.

Mindfulness involves both attitude and practice, and our ability to live mindfully grows with time. Some mindfulness practices are formal, such as seated meditation, while others are informal, more of a shift in attitude and focus while going about an ordinary action. Although the central attitude of mindfulness—acceptance of the current moment—is not always easy to carry out, especially when things aren't going your way, over time practitioners generally report a decrease in suffering.

Acceptance of the Moment

Acceptance of the moment doesn't mean you have to like what's happening or that all of your feelings are pleasant. It simply means being with what is.

There is a human tendency to run from pain and discomfort. We find so many ways to avoid it. We get out of balance and overdo activities that we hope will help us escape. For some, it's substance abuse—food, alcohol, or drugs—while for others, it's shopping, or too much TV, or too much gossip. It doesn't matter what the activity is. Most of these activities are fine in reasonable proportion and used appropriately. It's only when they become an escape hatch from the present that they become problematic and turn against us, robbing us of the very precious awareness that could alleviate our distress and bring us fullness in the joy of the moment.

exercise: Do You Try to Escape from Worry?

Do you ever find yourself coping with worry in any of the following ways? Do you find that you do the following? Answer yes or no after each item in the list.

- eat too much
- drink too much alcohol
- shop compulsively
- work compulsively
- retreat from people
- sleep too much
- watch more TV
- spend long, unproductive hours on your computer
- complain or gossip
- stay overly busy
- blame others

All of the above coping—or worry—styles are designed to help you avoid concerns and issues that you find troubling. While some of these do bring immediate relief, it's generally short lived.

Mindfulness asks that rather than moving away from your worries, you move toward them and hold them until they transform. The idea is to make friends with your issues rather than try to escape them. Like Max in the children's book *Where the Wild Things Are* (Sendak 1963), who found himself surrounded by monsters and overcame them by looking directly into their eyes, you look deeply at what is. You allow your monsters to be as they are and then you find peace, just as Max found himself back in his warm bed.

The practice of mindfulness encourages you to be present to everything in your life, just as it is in the moment. You learn to be present to your own experience, both the pleasurable and the challenging. Mindfulness might be noticing what troubles you, but it might also be noticing the beauty and fullness of a moment. It begins with learning to tune in and often involves slowing down to be able to notice what's actually there. It takes you into the present, the only place where you can really live, and away from worries about the future or regrets about the past.

All of the mind-body exercises in this book are to be practiced mindfully, meaning with focus, acceptance, and awareness of the moment. The breathing exercise that follows will introduce you to formal mindfulness practice.

Mindful Breathing

Mindful breathing is a core practice in mindfulness and a central practice in most meditative and stress-reduction approaches. To do this practice, you will want to find a place that is peaceful and beautiful, a place where you can be free of distractions.

exercise: Simple Mindful Breathing

Take the following steps to bring yourself into the present and into yourself.

1. Sit comfortably with an erect spine. You can sit on the floor or on a chair. It's also okay to do this exercise lying down, but if you have a tendency to fall asleep, you should do the exercise while seated.

2. Become aware of the breath. Notice it moving in and out. Notice the sensations of breathing and where you feel the breath. Perhaps you feel it in the nose, perhaps in the chest, perhaps in the belly.

3. Simply breathe while being aware of the breath rising and falling.

4. When thoughts come, let them come and then let them go, gently returning your attention to the breath. Remember, it's normal for the mind to think, so don't expect a totally still mind. Just come back to the breath.

Another way to practice mindful breathing is to repeat certain words or phrases silently to yourself as you watch your breath. For example, as you breathe in, you might say to yourself, "I am aware I am breathing in." As you breathe out, you might say to yourself, "I am aware I am breathing out" (Nhat Hanh 1993, 17). You simply continue breathing, thinking those simple words, watching the breath, and bringing yourself back to the breath and to these phrases whenever your mind wanders.

Your concentration and ease with breathing mindfully will grow over time if you make it a regular practice. After a while, you may come to consider the breath your home, where you—like Max at the end of *Where the Wild Things Are*—can feel safe, warm, and well fed.

Setting Your Intention

Mindful breathing can be part of a formal mind-body program. You will want to set your intention to practice regularly by finding a regular time in your schedule to do mindful breathing. It doesn't need to be a long time, and your practice space can be as simple as a cushion or chair in the corner of your bedroom or a pretty spot in your backyard. Having this regular time and place to practice will help you progress.

You can begin your formal practice of mindful breathing by setting five minutes aside at the beginning and gradually increasing it. You may want to consider practicing for as long as you can and then for one minute longer. In this way, your ability to maintain mindfulness will increase without undo strain.

Exercise: Setting Your Intention to Practice

Take a moment now to write down a good time and place for you to regularly practice mindful breathing.

____

____

You can change the time and place later, if necessary. The point is to make a commitment to breathe mindfully.

Congratulations. You have learned how to practice mindfulness to reduce your stress and have set an intention to do it regularly. Whether using CBT or mindfulness, or some combination of these two techniques, you are well on your way to conquering your worries.

Key Points

- It's normal to worry if you're having trouble conceiving.
- It's important to name and understand your fears.
- Noticing whether your worries are in the present or are about an unknown future may help you evaluate your worry. Worry is about the future, which is unknown.
- Understanding if you're a worrier may help you put your concerns in perspective.
- Cognitive behavioral therapy can help you evaluate and reframe your worried thoughts.
- Practicing mindfulness will help you be in the present and transform your experience.
- Mindful breathing is a central practice.

3

seeking medical help and coping with diagnosis and treatment

If you're having difficulty conceiving, at some point you probably will want to gather facts about fertility and about your body. In gathering facts, you will be better able to decide whether or not your concerns are justified and, most importantly, what you can do to remove obstacles to pregnancy.

The medical world defines infertility as one year of unsuccessful effort or, for women thirty-five and over, six months of unsuccessful effort. This is important to you in a couple of ways. First, if you're very worried and have been trying for a much shorter time than one year (or six months if you're over thirty-five), you most certainly have no need to be concerned yet. The official definition of infertility also may be important to you if you're counting on insurance reimbursement for your care, since many insurance companies will not reimburse some infertility-related procedures unless your attempts to become pregnant have been unsuccessful for a year (or six months if you're over thirty-five). This may or may not affect some of your early choices, but it's best to be aware of it and talk to your insurance company before you seek treatment.

This chapter outlines what to consider when choosing a fertility specialist. It will help you know what to expect if you go to a specialist and give you tools to organize and track your experience. The Taking Charge section focuses on journaling, a practice that can ease emotions and decrease the stress that can be associated with medical treatment.

Getting Started with a Fertility Specialist

If you've been trying on your own long enough to fit the official definition of infertility, if you've experienced more than one miscarriage, or if you have menstrual irregularities, you may be ready for a fertility workup. Your regular obstetrician-gynecologist (ob-gyn) may have experience with infertility and be able to perform an initial fertility evaluation, or she may refer you to a specialist. A fertility specialist, or *reproductive endocrinologist* (RE), is an ob-gyn who has completed at least two additional years of specialized training in infertility. Ultimately, the choice to see a specialist will be up to you. Some couples, depending on their personal and medical circumstances, decide to seek specialized help sooner than others.

When choosing a specialist, you will want to consider a range of factors, including success rate, procedures offered, doctor's experience, affordability (including whether your insurance is accepted), nonmedical services provided (such as counseling and mind-body work), geographical proximity, practice size, medical policies, and the general tone of the practice. Your regular doctor may be able to help you get started, but the better informed you are, the more comfortable you'll be in making a choice. What follows is a brief discussion of the various factors to consider.

Success Rate of the Practice

When you're looking for a fertility doctor, one of the first things you will want to know is the success rate of that doctor or medical practice. The Centers for Disease Control keeps statistics on the success rates of fertility practices on its website (see resources). Of course, you will want to find a practice with better-than-average outcomes. Note that if a practice treats women of all ages and conditions, its success rate might be lower than a practice that treats only couples with the highest chance of success. Therefore, if you are considering a particular practice, finding out what population it serves will give you more information about its real rate of success.

Procedures Offered

The websites for different medical practices usually include what procedures the practices offer. If you need additional information about a particular doctor or medical practice, someone in the office should be able to answer your questions.

Doctor's Experience

As you choose a doctor, consider the doctor's background, including educational and training background. How long has this doctor been in practice? Does the doctor have any special areas of expertise that might be important to you?

Affordability

Expenses will vary between medical practices, as will financial policies. Some practices may not be covered under your insurance (note that you should check to see if your health insurance covers infertility treatments). Some practices offer special packages or money back to some populations if treatments are unsuccessful. There may be a financial counselor on staff who can help you understand your options.

Nonmedical Services

Some medical practices offer onsite counseling, mind-body programs, and, as noted above, fertility-related financial counseling. These services may or may not be important to you. Many of these services can also be found outside of fertility practices. You may value having all these resources in one place or prefer to seek nonmedical support elsewhere.

Geographical Proximity

Fertility treatments can involve many visits to an office or clinic, and it's important to consider how accessible a specialist will be to you. Spending more travel time than necessary can add to your stress. If two clinics are similar in other ways, think about choosing the one that's easier for you to get to.

Size of Practice

Some medical practices consist of just a doctor or two, while others are very large. You may prefer a larger practice, where several doctors can back up one another, or a smaller, more intimate setting. If you choose a large practice, you will want to know if you'll be seeing the same doctor each time or not.

Medical Policies of Practice

Medical policies differ between practices. For example, if you're doing IVFs, you may want to know the policies regarding embryo transfer. Will you be able to choose how many embryos are transferred to you, or will the doctor decide? Some doctors have a policy of transferring a greater number of embryos than others. This may be an important consideration for you, since a higher number of embryos transferred can increase your chance of multiple births.

Personality of the Practice

You may get a feeling of the general tone of a medical practice during a visit or even through an initial phone call. Some settings are more friendly, supportive, and accessible than others. If a warm and supportive environment is important to you, you may be able to reduce your anxiety simply by choosing a practice with those qualities. On the other hand, the personality of the setting may be less important to you than other considerations. Once again, it's important to know yourself and honor your needs.

---

exercise: Identifying Your Priorities

Think about your own situation, including your medical needs, your personality, and your financial issues. Review the different factors covered in the previous section and then list your top priorities in choosing a fertility specialist.

____

____

____

____

____

Being aware of your priorities will help focus your search for the best specialist for you.

After you understand your priorities, you can begin doing your research. You may want to record your findings as you look into different medical practices or clinics specializing in infertility treatment.

exercise: Recording Your Research

Make several copies of the following blank worksheet so you can record information about each practice you're considering.

At the top of the worksheet, write the name of the practice you're researching, and then in the following categories record any information about it that you want to remember. Alternatively, you can rate the practice with a plus or a minus in each category. Be sure to compare your findings with your priorities.

Name of fertility clinic or practice: ______________________________

Success rate: ______________________________

Procedures offered: ______________________________

____

Doctor's experience: ______________________________

Affordability: ______________________________

Nonmedical services: ______________________________

Location: ______________________________

Size: ______________________________

Medical policies: ______________________________

Other considerations or impressions: ______________________________

____

Based on your research and your priorities, you should be able to choose the fertility practice or clinic that best meets your needs.

The Fertility Workup: Knowing What to Expect

If you have decided to see a reproductive endocrinologist, you will most likely undergo a standard diagnostic fertility workup plus any additional tests or procedures that seem to fit your circumstances. If you've already started to explore your fertility with your general ob-gyn, you'll want to provide the RE with your records, so that nothing is unnecessarily repeated.

The fertility workup gives you basic information about what's going on with your body, and you will probably want to rule out any obvious problems like blocked Fallopian tubes that can be addressed only once they're known. According to the Centers for Disease Control and Prevention (2011), in about a third of couples, the man is the infertile partner. So if you go to a fertility doctor, your partner will also be tested.

How Fertility Works

To understand the basic workup, it's helpful to know how fertility works. The female reproductive system includes the brain, the ovaries, the Fallopian tubes, and the uterus. Your doctor will evaluate these four aspects of your reproductive health over different stages of the menstrual cycle.

When a female child is born, she has all of the eggs that her body will ever produce. The eggs (*oocytes*) are found in fluid-filled sacs, known as *follicles*. Each menstrual cycle starts when the pituitary gland (located at the base of the brain) releases a hormone called *follicle stimulating hormone* (FSH). Over the first three to five days of the menstrual cycle, FSH stimulates the ovaries to make several follicles ready to release an egg. The ovarian cells start producing a variety of the hormone estrogen called *estradiol* (E2), which helps the chosen eggs start getting ready to be released. The FSH and E2 work in concert to stimulate egg development so that by cycle day eight or nine, one of the several chosen follicles becomes the leader. This is then the dominant follicle, which will mature and *ovulate* (release an egg).

Between days twelve and fourteen of the menstrual cycle, the pituitary gland releases yet another hormone, *luteinizing hormone* (LH). The LH surge is the trigger for ovulation to occur. The follicle at this stage measures between eighteen and twenty millimeters. The LH also stimulates the ovaries to produce the hormone *progesterone*, which prepares the lining of the uterus for implantation.

The egg moves out of the ovary and down the Fallopian tube toward the uterus. Sperm, which have been deposited in the vagina, swim up the female reproductive tract via the cervix, the uterus, and Fallopian tube. When the sperm and egg meet in the Fallopian tube, fertilization occurs. The early embryo develops for about three to five days in the Fallopian tube and then makes its way to the uterus and implants in its lining, where it develops until it is ready to be born.

If no sperm is present to fertilize the egg or if for any other reason no embryo gets implanted, the lining of the uterus then sloughs off. This is the first day of the next menstrual cycle.

If you are having fertility issues, it may be because one of these steps is not going exactly as described here. The doctor will check whether you are ovulating, whether you have sufficient eggs of good quality, and whether your hormone levels will support a pregnancy.

What follows are brief descriptions of fertility workups for women and men. You'll be able to find more detailed descriptions on your doctor's website or through Resolve (see resources). Your doctor is the best one to answer your questions.

Basic Fertility Workup for Women

A basic fertility workup will include a review of your medical history, a physical exam, testing for ovulation, testing for ovarian reserve, and testing your uterus and Fallopian tubes.

Medical History

Your doctor will likely start by taking a medical history. You will be asked your age, how long you've been trying to get pregnant, and whether you have had children before (having trouble getting pregnant when you were able to get pregnant before is called *secondary infertility*). Your doctor will also ask you about your menstrual history and any other medical issues you have, how often and when you have sex, whether you use lubricants, how much alcohol and caffeine you drink, and other questions. Some of these might feel a bit invasive but that are necessary for the doctor to fully understand the factors that may be affecting your fertility.

Physical Examination

The doctor will perform a complete physical exam. Among what will be assessed are your *body mass index* (BMI) (a calculation relating weight and height), evidence of increased hair growth, acne, and whether you are either overweight or underweight. The doctor will also do a pelvic exam along with a transvaginal ultrasound (TVUS) exam to make sure you don't have any anatomic difficulties such as fibroids or endometriosis.

Depending on your medical profile and the results of early testing, your doctor may perform additional tests and procedures. Your doctor is the one best equipped to explain the tests he or she will want to perform and why, but here are some of the most basic tests that you can expect as you get started.

Testing for Ovulation

You will want to know if and when you are ovulating. Even before you go to a specialist, your primary care doctor may suggest that you chart your *basal temperature* or use an over-the-counter *ovulation predictor kit*. To chart your basal temperature, you will take your temperature orally each morning the moment you awaken for at least a month and record the temperature daily. Normally, the release of progesterone due to ovulation causes a rise in temperature of 0.5 to 1.0 degree Fahrenheit. An ovulation predictor test is a urine test designed to detect the surge of luteinizing hormone that occurs about a day or day and a half before ovulation.

Testing for Ovarian Reserve

One of the major questions you will want to have answered is the condition of your ovaries. Remember that each woman is born with a finite (though very large) number of eggs, and we never make new eggs. We lose eggs both through ovulation and menstruation and through a natural process called atresia until we reach menopause, at which point we have depleted our store of functioning eggs. Also, as we age, our eggs become more prone to chromosomal abnormalities, which increase the risk of having children with genetic abnormalities such as Down syndrome. Fertility doctors try to assess *ovarian reserve*, how many eggs you have that could produce a viable pregnancy, as one of the first steps in determining egg quantity and quality. Your ovarian reserve can be determined by a combination of blood tests and sonograms.

Day-three follicle-stimulating hormone and estradiol testing. As discussed earlier, FSH and E2 are hormones involved in the process of stimulating the follicles to get ready to release eggs and stimulating eggs to mature for ovulation. FSH is produced in the pituitary gland in the brain, and it stimulates the follicles in the ovaries to mature. Once an egg starts to mature, it releases E2, which sends a message to the pituitary to stop sending more FSH. This suppression takes place by day three of your menstrual cycle. But if no eggs have matured to send out the E2 signal, the pituitary will just keep sending FSH, trying and trying to get an egg to mature.

By measuring both FSH and E2 levels on day three of your menstrual cycle, the doctor can get a pretty good indication of whether you have enough healthy eggs to get pregnant. The doctor may also do an ultrasound on day three to see how many follicles have been stimulated and are getting ready for action. Diminished ovarian reserve is generally diagnosed if your FSH levels are too high or your E2 levels are too high or too low and if fewer than eight follicles are developing.

These are not perfect tests, however. You can have normal hormone levels and still not have enough ovarian reserve. And though studies have shown that abnormal test results are a good predictor that the woman won't be able to get pregnant with her own eggs, in my practice, I have seen women with abnormal test results go on to conceive.

Clomid challenge. If you are over thirty-five, your doctor may prescribe the Clomid challenge to see if your pituitary gland and ovaries are talking to each other correctly. With the Clomid challenge, your doctor will first get day-three FSH and E2 levels but then challenge the ovaries by having you take Clomid, a fertility drug that should stimulate ovulation if enough good eggs are present, and then retesting the levels of FSH and E2 on day ten. Just as in the day-three test, an abnormal FSH or E2 level on day ten usually means not enough eggs have matured to send out E2, which makes it a indicator of poor ovarian reserve.

Testing Your Uterus and Fallopian Tubes

The best tools to see what's going on with your uterus and Fallopian tubes are X-ray and sonograph. The *hysterosalpingogram* (HSG) is a test designed to see if the inside of the uterus has a normal shape and whether there is an obstruction in the tubes. This test is done between days five and nine of your cycle and is usually performed in a hospital or radiology center, because the test involves X-rays. A dye that blocks X-rays is inserted into the uterine cavity through the cervix. The dye makes the shape of the uterus and Fallopian tubes show up brightly on the X-ray, which allows the doctor to determine whether there are any abnormalities, such as lesions, polyps, or fibroids, that might prevent a fertilized egg from implanting in the uterus or cause miscarriage, or whether the Fallopian tubes have any blockages that would keep an egg from making its way down them to the uterus.

A *sonohysterogram* (also called a *hysterosonogram*) is an ultrasound of the uterus performed after a small amount of salt water (saline solution) has been injected through the cervix into the vagina. The saline holds the walls of the uterus apart so the doctor can see the walls clearly in an ultrasound image. Then the doctor can see if your uterus has an abnormal shape or if there are growths of any kind that might interfere with implantation or cause miscarriage.

Basic Fertility Workup for Men

The male workup also starts with a medical history. The doctor will ask your partner whether he has fathered previous pregnancies, what medications he's used, whether he's had any sexually transmitted diseases, how much he exercises, and about his recreational drug use, among other things. The doctor will perform a physical exam and will order a semen analysis to check for sperm count, sperm *motility* (the ability of sperm to swim), *velocity* of the sperm (how fast they swim), *morphology* of the sperm (size and shape), and *liquefaction* of the semen (or its ability to go from a gel-like state at ejaculation to a liquid state inside your body). Your partner may also need to undergo hormonal testing to make sure his testicles are functioning properly.

Diagnosis

Once a general fertility workup is completed, your doctor may suggest more tests or procedures related to your particular situation. If problems are found during testing, those problems will form the basis of a diagnosis. It also may be that you fall into the 20 percent for whom no problems are found, and you are told that your infertility is unexplained. The various permutations of medical diagnoses and treatment options are best handled in conversation with your doctor, but additional general information is easily found online. To start, you may want to check the websites of Resolve or the American Society for Reproductive Medicine (see resources).

Reacting to Your Visits with the Doctor

If you're dealing with doctors and medical information, it's likely that you will have questions and worries. It's also possible that if you're stressed during a visit, you may not always hear information correctly.

You will feel more in charge and more organized if you can sort through your thoughts in a systematic way. One way is to keep a log of your visits, which you can add to as time passes. You can use this log before and after visits to help you remember what was said and to formulate your questions. You can use it in between visits to write down other questions you may have. You can even take it with you to record your doctor's answers. You may want to use a notebook, or you can use the chart in the next exercise.

exercise: Question Log

Make multiple copies of the following worksheet and use it to log the dates of your visits, questions you have, and the answers you receive from your doctor or doctors.

Date of Visit	Your Questions	Doctor's Answers

Choosing your RE wisely, understanding tests and procedures, and communicating your questions to your doctor will help you feel more in charge and may help you achieve your best possible fertility outcome.

Comparing Your Worries with Medical Information

Once you've gone to a doctor, you will have medical input that may be very encouraging or totally devastating; for most, it's somewhere in the middle. Even if you are in the 20 percent whose infertility is unexplained by test results, you will have ruled out some possibilities and in that way will have more information than you had before. Your medical situation will also be evaluated and reevaluated over time, based on your reactions to tests and procedures.

What can be upsetting or simply confusing about test results is that most doctors will speak to you in terms of your statistical odds of becoming pregnant. When presented with statistics, it's important to remember that you are an individual and not a statistic. Statistical odds are just that, statistical odds. In fact, the odds your doctor gives you may be on the low side of your real potential, since they don't account for the impact of practicing mind-body techniques. You're working in this book because you know that mind-body practices, the very practices you're learning, have repeatedly been demonstrated to significantly increase a woman's chance of becoming pregnant (Domar et al. 2000; Domar and Nikolovski 2009).

In the years I have been working with infertility, I've seen many examples of women working with mind-body approaches being told they had little or even no chance of becoming pregnant. Many went on to have babies. A few examples may be encouraging. In one mind-body group for fertility, two of the eight women in the group were given a zero percent chance of pregnancy by their doctors. Both went on to become pregnant during the course of the group. Another who was told her chances were grim went on to adopt and very soon thereafter became pregnant and gave birth. Jessica, whose story you'll read next, was one of the most surprising and inspirational of the women I've worked with. She had given up.

Jessica's Story

Jessica was told her eggs were too old and that there was no way she could conceive a child using her own eggs. After several failed IVFs, she became convinced this was the case. Jessica decided to try an IVF with donor eggs, a procedure that could dramatically increase her chance of pregnancy.

Jessica selected a donor and went through a donor egg IVF cycle. She got pregnant but miscarried early in the pregnancy. Determined, Jessica tried a second donor IVF. This time, she did not conceive. After several years of effort, Jessica and her doctor gave up on the hope that she could conceive and carry a pregnancy even with donor eggs.

Jessica grieved the loss of a dream, but ever the survivor, she began thinking of her other options: adoption or child-free living. Adoption, she reasoned, could come later if she and her husband decided that's what they wanted to do. After all, she did enjoy life with her husband and her career. Gradually she began to accept the idea of not having any biological children and of not adopting in the near future, and gradually the pleasure of living returned. She continued the healthy habits that she had developed during the time she was trying to conceive—eating well, exercising moderately, practicing mindfulness meditation, seeing her acupuncturist, and working out personal issues in psychotherapy. Jessica was in her mid-forties when she called to tell me that she had given birth to a healthy baby girl, surprisingly and unexpectedly conceived the old-fashioned way.

Your situation may or may not be anything like Jessica's or the women I described earlier who were given grim prognoses and yet became pregnant. On the other hand, you may be very like them. Is there a reason to believe you aren't? They are real women who had good outcomes in spite of scary statistics. Although scientific understanding of the factors that contribute to fertility continues to grow, there is still some mystery and speculation, and in the space between fact and mystery lies possibility.

Choosing Mind-Body Practices Alone or Combined with Medical Treatment

Some couples decide that they don't want to pursue Western medical fertility procedures until after they have given other approaches a try, while others use mind-body approaches as a complement to treatment. This is a very personal choice and depends on your temperament and beliefs, your physical status, including your age, and your trust and commitment to any course you choose. For example, if you're young and have no known problems that would predict infertility but know you've had a high stress level and an unhealthy lifestyle, it may make a lot of sense to spend some time working with mind-body techniques before embarking on any treatment. On the other hand, just as a hypothetical, if you're pushing against age limits and your doctor is suggesting you try in vitro fertilization, you may want to combine medical treatment with a mind-body program right away.

Taking Charge: Journaling

To deal with infertility is to deal with a multitude of emotions, facts, questions, appointments, and decisions. Journaling can be a comforting and healing way to ride out the storm. Journaling can help you clarify and record thoughts, release and transform feelings, and even make your body healthier.

The Positive Effects of Journaling

James Pennebaker, a psychology professor and researcher at the University of Texas, in a series of now well-known experiments has documented the positive effects of journaling on both mood and health. Pennebaker asked many groups of people from all walks of life to write about traumatic events in their lives or the worst things that had happened to them. They were asked to write for fifteen minutes at a time for four days. What he discovered was that as difficult emotions were released through journaling, both mood and immune function improved (2002), and people who wrote about traumatic events had fewer doctor visits for the next six weeks than those who wrote only about trivial events (Pennebaker, Keicolt-Glaser, and

Glaser 1988). In the same study, Pennebaker drew blood from the participants and was able to demonstrate an increase in the cells that fight disease. This is especially interesting since the same autonomic nervous system that impacts immune function also impacts hormone function. We can speculate that if the release of emotions through journaling can impact the immune system, it may also impact the very hormones needed for reproduction.

Whether or not you believe that journaling will boost your fertility, expressing emotions can definitely boost your mood and help you feel better while dealing with your fertility issues.

Using Journaling to Cope with Difficult Emotions

Holding in difficult emotions from past and current events takes effort. Releasing those emotions with words, whether written or spoken, can relieve the burden on mind and body, allowing for greater overall well-being.

Coping with any level of a fertility issue will produce many difficult feelings and thoughts, and releasing emotions can become more important during this time than it may have been in the past. Many women with fertility problems feel disconnected from formerly close friends. Many of your friends may not have experienced difficulty with fertility, and they may not be people with whom you can share your deepest feelings. You may even feel that your generally supportive partner either doesn't truly understand what you're experiencing or has become tired of discussing fertility issues. Having an outlet for emotions in the form of a journal, where you can write freely and privately about your deepest concerns, can be an important and helpful component of your mind-body program and your overall sense of wellness.

There are many ways to journal and many purposes for doing so. You may journal to release difficult emotions as discussed above, to organize your thoughts, or to keep track of your appointments, questions, and mind-body practice. You may journal to express yourself creatively either with words or drawing. Your journal, however you use it, can be a wonderful companion.

If you choose to use your journal to address difficult emotions, you may want to use one of the approaches below. Whichever approach you choose, remember, the beginning of this exercise can and should open painful emotions, which is not the same as creating stress. Your feelings are already there. Acknowledging and releasing your feelings will ultimately reduce, not increase, your stress. It is the effort of suppressing these feelings that produces stress on both body and mind. As is often the case in healing, you may feel temporarily worse, but ultimately you should feel better. If this, for any reason, doesn't seem true for you after some experimentation, please listen to your own inner wisdom about how you can best use your journal.

exercise: Writing about Past Trauma

If you want to follow the Pennebaker protocol, write for fifteen minutes at a time for four consecutive days about the worst things in your life. These could be things that happened in your childhood or at any time in your life. Allow your thoughts and emotions to flow. Don't worry about grammar, spelling, or anything other than writing. Keep going. Journaling in this way, being present to your experience, is something like staying present to your experience in mindfulness. It's a way to embrace experience—what actually is—rather than escaping it, and a way to allow uncomfortable experience to transform. The relief comes not when the wound is first opened but after it has had some time to heal.

You can use the same protocol of writing for fifteen minutes for four consecutive days while limiting your writing to a particular topic that is painful or difficult.

exercise: Writing about Infertility

Write about infertility for four sessions. Do this just as you would if you were writing about old traumas, as in the previous exercise, except that the focus is on infertility or your fears of infertility. Again, don't worry about how the quality of the writing or how it looks on the page. Simply express your thoughts and feelings.

Another way to address your feelings about infertility is to have a dialogue with infertility in a straightforward, head-on way. This will help you to review your experience and air your feelings, hopes, and fears, speaking directly to the cause.

exercise: Have a Dialogue with Infertility

Imagine that infertility is an unwelcome guest, a kind of entity or being that has come to visit, and you are having a conversation with it. To do this, imagine that Infertility is like a person, born at a particular time and place and dressed in a particular way. Now create a dialogue between yourself and Infertility as if you were in a play or a novel. Write down the dialogue in your journal, and act out both roles so that you are the voice of Infertility as well as yourself.

That's an exercise that you may want to try now and again later in your journey. Your relationship with infertility will change over time. The dialogue will give you a way to check in with yourself and what you feel you're up against.

Keeping a regular journal can also be a good way to release your emotions and avoid stuffing your feelings. As you express your feelings, you will feel less burdened.

exercise: Writing about Current Issues

Keep an ongoing journal about what's going on in your daily life, especially the emotional issues that arise in your relationships—with your partner, your friends, and your colleagues at work—as well as your ongoing emotions surrounding your fertility. Do this as a part of your regular mind-body program.

As you keep a record of your thoughts, you may find that you tend to ruminate on them less. If you have found it hard to concentrate on things other than your fertility issues, having a place for your thoughts and feelings can help free you to enjoy the other parts of your life.

Additional Ideas for Journaling

Not all useful journaling is about the emotional difficulties in life. Some other kinds of journaling—such as keeping a gratitude journal, drawing in your journal, or writing poetry in your journal—can be equally beneficial.

A gratitude journal is a fabulous way to keep an appreciation of what is good in your life while dealing with infertility. Writing every day about five things for which you're grateful can help you shift your focus away from what is wrong, or potentially wrong, toward what is working well. You can write in your gratitude journal whenever you like, or you may want to use it at the beginning or end of other mind-body practices.

Drawing is an activity that can help you bypass linear thought processes and creatively integrate deeply felt emotions. You don't need to be an artist to keep a drawing journal. You can use markers, pens, chalk, or whatever implements you choose to let whatever presents itself take form. You may even want to try drawing with your nondominant hand: if you're right-handed, try drawing with your left hand, or vice versa. This can help you access parts of the brain that you don't reach when using your dominant hand and also remind you that drawing really doesn't need to be about being artistic. Of course, if you happen to be an artist, you can also use your journal as a place to exercise your skill and express your feelings.

Writing poetry in your journal, as with drawing, is about allowing your ideas to flow without worrying too much about quality. This is about moving outside your rational linear mental processes and accessing hidden parts of your being. If poetry scares you, you may want to look up some simple poetry forms—haiku is a good one—that you can use as a guide. But remember, it's not about following rules but about allowing your creative side to help you release your emotions.

Many people thrive on journaling. I hope you will find a way to make it work for you. However you use it, try to write something, even if it's very short, every day. A journal can be a wonderful companion.

Key Points

- Evaluating your infertility concerns will at some point involve seeing a doctor.
- When choosing your doctor, you will need to consider your priorities and do research.
- A basic fertility workup includes tests for you and your partner.
- Statistics are important but not always predictive of your result.
- Journaling is a valuable mind-body practice for managing the emotions that go along with infertility and its treatment.

4

the emotional roller coaster

Dealing with infertility has been likened to riding a roller coaster. One minute you're hoping for a baby. Perhaps you tune to your body and it just *feels* pregnant. Your breasts feel full; your period is late. You start choosing names. You picture yourself holding your baby, bringing her home, showing her to friends and family. The next moment, you find that you're not pregnant. You get your period or learn that an IVF didn't work. You've fallen from the peak, the top of the roller coaster track, to the bottom, and you probably feel the emotional equivalent of the stomach dropping that you might feel on an actual roller-coaster ride.

But, just as in a roller-coaster ride, you don't stay in one place very long. You're going to try again, and so you need to quickly move past your disappointment and hope that things will go better in the next cycle. You try again, this time perhaps with the assistance of a new fertility protocol, and you hope this will be the time that your dreams come true. The roller coaster starts moving up the track again, and if you don't succeed this time, the drop from hope to disappointment can be ever more precipitous and painful. This rapid cycling of hope and disappointment can make for a dizzying and difficult emotional ride.

This chapter will help you understand that ride and provide you with strategies to help you cope. It will encourage you to review and evaluate your personal fertility roller coaster. As always, understanding your own experience will be the starting point for finding personal solutions. The Taking Charge section will introduce you to some meditation techniques for helping you steady your ride.

Understanding the Ride: Why Infertility Is So Emotionally Challenging

Infertility can cause an intense and complicated mix of feelings. You probably feel many things at the same time or at different times—happy expectation, sadness, anger, envy—and it's very difficult to handle emotions that change frequently. Understanding why this time is so difficult can help you find compassion for yourself and strategies to help you manage. Here are some of the reasons it can be so hard. You may find that some of these apply to you more than others.

You must adjust to quickly changing circumstances. You don't know what to expect, and you must rapidly adjust your emotions and planning to fit new information. There are many ups and downs, twists and turns, calling for emotional responses and often for practical decision-making as well.

All areas of life can be affected and must be managed. Infertility can impact your body, your relationships, your finances, your social life, your time management, and your overall life planning. Knowing when or if to buy a house, change a job, or even plan a vacation can be dependent on whether or not you become pregnant. You may decide to head in one direction, and then something occurs that makes you reverse course. You may feel you're in limbo waiting for your fertility issues to resolve before you can move forward.

The stress of infertility is cumulative. In the beginning, you hope for pregnancy to just happen naturally. If it doesn't happen, you may follow a progression from no problem to possible problem to problem that needs intervention. If you work with a fertility specialist and are using assisted reproductive technology (ART), the intervention may progress from the less invasive to the more invasive or extreme. Intrauterine insemination (IUI), when unsuccessful, is often followed by in vitro fertilization. So as time passes, you may feel that the stakes are getting higher. You may have a certain number of IVFs that you can or are willing to try. Age sometimes becomes a factor because of changes in your body that make you less fertile or because of policies of the fertility practice to do IVFs only with women under a certain age. Choices such as the decision to use donor eggs or surrogates may present themselves. Over time, some couples face difficult choices about when to quit and save their financial and emotional resources for alternative family building options, such as adoption. It may feel that the harder and longer you try, the more stressed you feel.

Infertility involves loss and grief. The experience of infertility involves loss even if ultimately you end up with a happy family. If you hoped that having a baby would be the result of an intimate evening with your partner, followed by a joyful announcement and celebration, any problem with conception or pregnancy constitutes a loss. It's the loss of an expected experience and most likely the loss of a dream. And, of course, thinking you might be pregnant and finding out that you're not, or having a miscarriage, is an even bigger loss. Yet grieving for your loss may be complicated. For one, your loss may be invisible to others, since they might not know about this personal part of your life. Those who do know about it may not understand and may minimize your feelings by telling you to just relax or to adopt or not to worry because it will eventually happen. Even your partner may minimize your feelings, due either to a lack of understanding or a desire to be supportive and encouraging. If this happens, you may feel very alone just when you most need support. Making all of this harder may be that you lack a ritual to help with your grief. Normally, if you were to lose someone in your life, there would be a funeral, a memorial, a sharing of memories, but if you lose a hoped-for pregnancy or an actual pregnancy, you may feel that someone has died and yet there is no shared ritual.

Hormonal changes can make emotions more intense. Most fertility treatments involve the manipulation of your hormones, which can lead to emotional volatility for some people. Just at the time when you're being stressed by concerns related to your fertility, you may be physiologically less steady and less able to weather the stress.

You may expect a lot of yourself. In spite of the stress that comes with infertility, you may feel that you should handle everything better than you are. You want to be optimistic for the next cycle. You most likely have responsibilities in your life, such as a job, that continue regardless of what's happening with your fertility. If you're feeling stressed, it may be more difficult to concentrate and to manage all that's on your plate.

Your self-esteem may suffer. Although infertility is a medical condition, you may feel that you're failing in some way each time you get disappointing news. If you're not feeling good about yourself, it is certainly more difficult to maintain a balanced emotional and personal life in challenging times. Just when you need self-understanding, you may be feeling self-judgmental and emotionally depleted.

You may judge yourself for having difficult emotions. You may also be like many women I've met who are judgmental about their feelings. It's not pleasant to feel anger and envy, and if you've learned to think of these as negative or bad feelings, you may be uncomfortable with yourself for having them, even though they are natural and experienced by most women who struggle with infertility.

Whatever complex feelings you have, you really can cope with them. This is an unpleasant and difficult time, but with mind-body practices and the support of your doctors, you will come out on the other side. Marianne did.

Marianne's Story

In her first therapy session, Marianne was so overwhelmed that it was difficult for her to stop crying long enough to tell her story. She had started trying to conceive after a wonderful first year of marriage, which she and her husband had decided to preserve for themselves as a couple before starting their family. That was three years earlier. Since that time, she had hoped every month that she would become pregnant, only to be disappointed every month. She had gone to her regular ob-gyn, who had told her she was fine and to just keep trying, for sometimes it takes a little time. After eleven more months of repeated disappointments, Marianne went to see a specialist, who was very encouraging. She tried IUIs and then IVFs. Nothing worked. Every failed cycle represented a major loss for her. Her mother didn't understand why she was trying so hard to have a biological child and advised her to adopt. As a result, there was now tension in the family as well.

By the time she arrived in my office, she was so exhausted by repeated disappointments that she felt she was a totally different person from who she was when she had married four years earlier, and she was concerned about the negative impact her emotional upset was having on her marriage, her work, and the other important relationships in her life. The final straw was that her doctor was now telling her that, at age thirty-eight, her egg quality was declining and she should consider trying a cycle with donor eggs. Marianne felt alone and defeated. She had been on an unusually difficult emotional roller coaster for too long, and she couldn't see how to help herself out of the hole into which she had fallen.

Marianne and I worked together for almost nine months. During that time, she was able to express her feelings, develop better ways of coping, and ultimately clarify her options and come up with the best solutions for herself and her husband.

Marianne had to give up on her hope of having a fully biological baby, but she was able to conceive using a donor egg. She experienced pregnancy, birth, breast feeding, and bonding with her baby from the very start. Despite the use of a donor egg, she knew this was her baby, truly her baby, and in a letter to me following the birth of her son, which included photos of her beautiful baby, she told me how happy she was as a mother and thanked me for helping her through a dark period in her life.

Back when she was on the emotional roller coaster, she would never have believed that she would find happiness if she couldn't have a baby with her own eggs, but once off the emotional roller coaster and in her new role as mom, she became happy and satisfied. During the course of her journey toward motherhood, she learned a lot about herself, her needs, and her possibilities.

Some of the issues Marianne explored in therapy and the strategies she developed are included in the exercises below. As you work with them, I hope they will help you, like Marianne, find greater understanding, peace, and clarity.

exercise: Exploring How Infertility Has Been Emotionally Difficult

Answer the following questions to reveal how coping with infertility has been difficult for you. If the topic of a question seems unrelated to your emotional difficulties, skip to the next question.

1. What information have you gathered about your fertility that has caused you to have to rapidly change your expectations, plans, or treatment? How have you reacted emotionally to these changes?

   ____

   ____

   ____

   ____

2. List the areas of your life that your fertility issues have had an impact on. How have your fertility issues impacted your ability to manage time, finances, and relationships? Think about how

your fertility issues have created emotional or practical ups and downs in each of these areas. Have you had to change your plans in any of these areas? What happened? How were you affected?

3. Has stress associated with infertility been cumulative? Compare yourself now with where you were emotionally at the beginning of your experience with infertility or possible infertility. How did you feel at the beginning of this journey? How did you feel at different times? What have been some of the highs and lows? How do you feel now?

4. In what ways have you experienced loss? Have you been able to grieve your loss? What kind of support do you have when you feel sad about a disappointment? Do you have any rituals to help you honor and resolve your sense of loss?

5. If you're in treatment that involves the use of hormones or the manipulation of your hormones with medications, how do you react to those hormones? What changes do you experience? If

you're not in treatment, have you had any issues with hormonal changes such as premenstrual syndrome (PMS) or hormonal changes around a miscarriage?

6. What are your self-expectations? Do you think that you should be able to handle everything better than you are? Do your expectations seem reasonable to you when you consider them calmly?

7. How has infertility impacted your sense of who you are? Has your self-esteem suffered?

8. Are you accepting of your feelings, or do you judge them and think that some of them are bad?

____

____

____

____

Practical Coping Strategies

Now that you've explored the emotional roller coaster that you experience around infertility, here are some coping strategies that can help you weather the ride.

Responding to Your Changing Circumstances

You can make a big difference in how you respond to change if you pay close attention to what's happening and give yourself credit for getting through it. Here are some basic rules to follow:

- Appreciate yourself for responding to change even when difficult.
- Note the times when change has been positive or beneficial.
- Gather the most accurate and complete information about your fertility, to allow yourself to feel confident about your options and best solutions.
- Use the mind-body techniques you are learning to feel more centered in spite of uncertainty.

In times of changing or unpredictable circumstances, it's also important to have some parts of your life that feel constant, reassuring, and predictable. It could be pizza on Friday nights, walking the dog at a certain time of day, taking a class, or going to a social or athletic event that occurs predictably. It could be a certain time and place to practice relaxation and meditation techniques.

exercise: Creating Consistency

List those activities in your life that are predictable and pleasant for you, those things that you can count on in the midst of change. Make these activities a regular part of life. In times when you are feeling shaky, remember to consult your list and reassure yourself that there are things in your life you can rely on.

____

____

____

____

Managing the Affected Areas of Your Life

You will feel more grounded if you look carefully at the areas of your life that are affected by your fertility issues and make small, positive changes in them. Here are some suggestions that may help:

- Strengthen your relationships by learning to know your needs and communicate them effectively to your partner, friends, and family.
- Meet with your personal financial advisor or a financial advisor at the fertility practice to decide on the best options for your situation. Be realistic about your resources and plan accordingly.
- Think through what stresses you have at work, and make plans to reduce these stresses or at least to put them in perspective.
- Reevaluate your long-term plans. Work with your partner to make sure that whatever plans you have at present aren't adding to your stress.

exercise: Taking Small Steps

Consider the impact of your fertility issues on your life. Which areas of your life are the most affected? Which the least? Try to think of one small way that you can improve an area that's significantly affected. If you can find even one small way to improve one area of your life, congratulate yourself. By taking one step in this one area, you are shifting into a solution-oriented mind-set, which will help you find more solutions in the future.

____

____

____

____

Coping with Your Cumulative Stress

As new stress piles on top of old stress, you can become emotionally exhausted or even depressed. Here are some tips for coping with cumulative stress:

- Recognize the cumulative nature of stress, and realize that over time you may become tired, just as you would if you were running a marathon.
- Consciously track your own reserves, so you know when you're running out of fuel.
- Find pleasurable activities that can restore your energy and help you appreciate your life.
- Consider taking a break from treatment if doing so wouldn't be a problem medically.
- Limit the amount of time you spend discussing fertility issues with your partner so that the more pleasurable aspects of your relationship can be kept alive.

Sometimes you may not consciously note the things that make you feel renewed, so having a list available can help.

exercise: Finding Activities That Renew You

List some activities that make you feel good. They can be anything from reading a book to going for a walk, doing yoga, watching a movie, talking to a friend, or taking a scented bath.

___

___

___

___

Try to do one or more of these activities each week. If you're having a difficult time, return to this list for ideas about what you can do to feel better.

Coping with Your Loss and Grieving

Grieving is an important part of life. If you experience a loss, don't push it aside. Instead, allow yourself to grieve. Here are some tips on grieving:

- Honor your loss. Take time to grieve.
- Be gentle to yourself.
- Create a ritual to help you grieve. A ritual can be something very simple that is meaningful to you, like writing a letter to a baby you lost or going for a walk with your partner and sharing your feelings about what has occurred.
- Create a community that you can talk with. Join a local support group or find one online.
- Explore the resources offered by Resolve (see resources).

exercise: Writing about Your Loss

Take time to write about the ways you might deal with loss. Do you have one or more people whom you trust to truly understand your feelings and support you? Can you think of a ritual that you could perform to honor your loss?

____

____

____

____

Simply writing about your feelings and acknowledging the resources that you have can help you cope with loss.

Handling Your Hormones

If you're in treatment, your hormones are affecting your mood and affecting your view of the world. Here are some ways to cope:

- Remind yourself frequently that some of your feelings are stronger now than they will be later, when your hormones are back to normal.
- Experiment with the idea that a strong emotion does not prove anything factual about you, another person, a situation, or the world.
- See if you can just notice the emotion without making it be about something.
- Ahead of time, agree on a signal to give your partner that indicates you're feeling emotional and tells your partner what you need. You could even incorporate humor. (*Hormone attack! Go away.* Or *Hormone attack! I need a hug.*)
- Think of the hormones as part of what's going to help you become a mother. Be gentle, compassionate, and understanding with yourself.

- Give yourself permission to avoid situations that might be upsetting and to focus on nurturing, soothing activities. Remind yourself that you're going through a lot and need to care for yourself.

exercise: Avoiding Stressful Activities

List the activities or people in your life that you associate with stress, and ask yourself if you can avoid them. If the answer is yes, then write down how you will avoid them, and choose to do so.

Stressful Activities or People	**Avoidable (Y/N)**	**How You Will Avoid Them**

If you're not sure that you can avoid a particular activity, ask yourself what would happen if you didn't show up and how bad that might be. Remember, although you want to be careful with the feelings of people who are important in your life, you especially need to focus on taking care of yourself at this time.

Addressing Your High Self-Expectations

If you have very high expectations of yourself, you may find yourself disappointed in your own behavior. If this is true for you, your idea of how you think you should be may be unrealistic. It's not easy dealing with infertility, and you're doing what you can to have a child. The following strategies can help you feel better.

- Appreciate your ability to persist in spite of many challenges.
- Tell yourself that this is a very unusual and challenging time in your life and that you are doing the best you can.
- Remember that sometimes it's only the hormones talking.
- Notice all the times you have overcome challenges, adjusted to change, and done what was necessary for your fertility and in the rest of your life.
- Be aware that dealing with infertility is very difficult for everyone and it's normal to react to stress.
- Connect with others in your situation.
- Release yourself from the need to be perfect.
- Focus on the positive.
- Notice your victories, even the small ones.
- Let go of shoulds.
- Congratulate yourself for all your efforts to have a child.

You've no doubt overcome many difficulties, and you deserve to appreciate yourself for that. There are many times when you have risen to the occasion. It may have been showing up for an appointment that was causing anxiety. It may have been managing a situation at work or with your family. It may have been something as simple as handling your emotions during a trip to the store, where you saw many mothers with young children. Recalling when you've done well with these situations can be a positive exercise.

exercise: Congratulating Yourself

Make a list of the times you dealt well with difficult situations, and congratulate yourself. Dealing well means having the courage and determination to get through the tough times. It doesn't mean having no feelings. Enter your own name in the first blank space and describe what you accomplished in the second.

Congratulations, ______________________ for, ______________________________________

____

Congratulations, ______________________ for, ______________________________________

____

Congratulations, ______________________ for, ______________________________________

____

Congratulations, ______________________ for, ______________________________________

____

Congratulations, ______________________ for, ______________________________________

____

You can add to the list as time goes by. In this way you will develop the habit of noticing the positive and appreciating yourself.

Confronting Your Low Self-Esteem

It's common for women dealing with infertility to struggle with self-esteem issues. Here are some coping strategies.

- Tell yourself that you are not defined by your fertility.
- Make a list of all your valued characteristics and accomplishments.
- Remember that you are dealing with something that is not your fault any more than needing glasses or contact lenses might be your fault.
- Do the things you're good at and that make you feel good about yourself.
- Surround yourself with people who value and love you.
- Practice the mind-body exercises that help you connect with your deeper self.

It's important to focus on what you like about yourself, what others value in you, and on your accomplishments. None of this changes in response to a fertility issue, but if fertility is taking center stage, you may forget to notice your strengths.

exercise: Focusing on Your Strengths

Take time now to list some things that make you feel good about yourself. Notice which thoughts, people, and activities make you feel good about yourself, and plan to increase them.

____

____

____

____

____

Tackling Your Self-Judgment

It's unrealistic to think that you will have only happy, generous feelings all the time when dealing with emotional challenges. Feelings such as envy or anger are common. Yet you may be judging yourself for having these difficult feelings. If you are, try the following coping strategies.

- Recognize that all feelings exist for a reason and are neither good nor bad in themselves.
- Some feelings are more pleasant than others. Remind yourself that it's part of the human experience to have a full range of feelings, not only pleasant, happy ones.
- Read books on this subject and talk to others who can validate your experience. You will see that you are only human.
- Use mind-body practices to feel better about yourself. As you do, you will be more at peace with yourself and others.
- Notice that when you feel anger or envy, it's only the flipside of your longing for a child. It's really not about the other person.
- Be compassionate with yourself whenever you can. You're doing the best you can.

If you're judging yourself for having certain thoughts and feelings, you are most likely your own harshest critic. And you may not have shared your feelings with anyone. If this is the case, you're listening only to your own inner critic. Sharing your emotions with another person who can support and reassure you can help you develop compassion for yourself. You can also imagine a perfectly wise, loving person who understands and loves you.

exercise: Learning to Be Compassionate with Yourself

Discuss your self-judgment with a real or imaginary person who does not judge you but supports and reassures you. Listen carefully to what this person says to you. Use the space below to write down the reassurances you receive.

Whenever you find yourself judging yourself, you can refer to this list. It will remind you how to show compassion to yourself. Then you can replace your harsh self-judging thoughts with the support and reassurance that you need.

Taking Charge: Meditation

Your most overarching complaint as you deal with your personal infertility roller coaster may be that so many things are out of your control. Try as you might to take care of yourself, try as you might to maintain a steady and optimistic attitude, that roller coaster keeps taking you around curves you hadn't expected and presenting you with new challenges. At times, when things don't go the way you would like, you may find yourself falling into a dark emotional pit that leaves you at odds with yourself and your world. At other times, a disappointment may inspire you to reach deeper and higher, to harness all of your internal and external resources to become your best possible self.

The practice of meditation can strengthen your ability to cope with fertility issues, helping you steady yourself on the emotional roller coaster. First, you must accept that with fertility, as with life in general, there are things that are out of your control. Recognizing and accepting this, you can learn to work with what you can control, your own thoughts and emotions, your own mind. Meditation is an ancient but contemporary tool to help you do just that. Developing a meditation practice now is one way to turn crisis to opportunity. Besides being a truly fulfilling way to steady your ride, meditation can also make for a happier, healthier you throughout your life.

Understanding Meditation

Meditation is about focus, concentration, and the training of the mind. The object of focus changes according to the style and philosophy of the specific meditation practice. There are many schools of meditation, but most people divide meditation into two main camps: concentrative meditations that emphasize concentration on a mantra or an object and mindfulness practices that focus more on sensation and being present to moment-to-moment experience, such as the mindful breathing practice suggested in chapter 2.

In this section, you will find a variety of meditation techniques from both camps and suggestions about how you can integrate meditation into your life. The important thing is to find the meditation techniques that work best for you—the ones you will practice. Whichever you choose, it's important to understand that meditation, although associated with Eastern religions, can be practiced with no religious content and is perfectly compatible with whatever religion you do practice or with the practice of no religion at all.

Concentrative Meditation

As the name implies, concentrative meditation involves focusing on one thing, such as a mantra or repetitive phrase. The concentration is intended to still the chatter of the mind and so allow for peace, clarity, and a deeper way of knowing yourself and the world. At the beginning, when you first begin to practice, you will probably find that your mind is very busy with many thoughts and concerns. This is normal and does not mean that you can't meditate. It's the mind's job to think, so there's no need to be distressed when it does its job. The Buddhists use the term *monkey mind* to describe the mind's tendency to move from thought to thought like a chattering monkey swinging from branch to branch. When you notice the activity of your mind, the trick is to accept that you are thinking, be loving with yourself, and gently return your attention to the breath and to the object of your concentration. Eventually, you might become aware that you are not your thoughts, and you might come to identify with the more enduring part of you that witnesses your thoughts as they come and go.

As you practice this, it may help for you to think of your thoughts as clouds passing by. Or you can think of them as e-mails coming in. You can see that they're there, but you don't need to open them and give them a lot of attention. Another useful metaphor is that of the ocean with its turbulent waves on the surface and its deep stillness below. The fact that you find turbulence on your surface in the form of many thoughts does not mean that you lack a place of stillness in your depths. Meditation, especially when practiced over time, can help you find the deep stillness within yourself.

The exercises that follow will give you an opportunity to experiment with different objects of concentration. See how each of these practices works for you. You may want to try one for several weeks and then switch to another, paying attention to how each one affects you over a little bit of time. If you're new to meditation, you may want to begin with five to fifteen minutes of meditation and gradually increase the time you spend. Begin each practice session by taking several deep, centering breaths.

Mantra Meditation

Mantra meditation is a traditional form of meditation in which a *mantra*, or a word or phrase, becomes the object of concentration. If you practice yoga or are drawn to the use of a traditional mantra, you may want to experiment with *Om Nama Shivaya* or *Hamsa* or another that you've encountered. In yoga traditions, some of these sounds are said to carry a vibration that can help you move into meditation.

Most of the people I work with, however, choose to find a personally meaningful word to use as their mantra, and for many this seems to be an excellent way to meditate, for the mantra elicits the qualities symbolized by the chosen focus word or phrase. A personally meaningful focus word can help you become one with an uplifting or steadying thought, feeling, or quality during the time that you're dealing with fertility issues and beyond.

The first step is to find the word or phrase that works for you. The words you use may change over time, and that's okay. On the other hand, you may find words that work for you over a long time. When you find an uplifting, steadying focus, you have a mental home and a spiritual shelter to return to whenever you like. There will be no more need to stand helplessly in the rain when you have such a home.

exercise: Practicing with a Mantra or Focus Word

Take a few moments to relax and search for your focus word or words. There is no right or wrong choice of focus words beyond determining whether your focus works for you. It may be obvious to you, but if you're like most of the people I've worked with on this exercise, a few moments of quiet reflection are in order.

Take several deep breaths. Fill your lungs completely. Allow your breath to deepen until you feel your abdomen expanding with each inhalation and relaxing inward with each exhalation. You may put your hands on your belly to see if this is happening.

To help you find a meaningful word or phrase, you may want to ask yourself these questions as you breathe, and see what floats into your awareness:

- What do you love?
- What would you like to feel?
- What qualities would you like to have?
- What do you find beautiful?
- What makes you feel safe?
- What makes you feel hopeful?
- What makes you happy?

Contemplate your answers to these questions. Do any of your answers suggest a word or phrase that you might like to use as a focus of meditation? Did something else arise that was not connected to these questions? Here are some words used by others: "trust," "love," "god," "relaxed," "calm," "trusting," "hope," "patience," "I am at peace," "I am at ease."

Once you've chosen your focus word or phrase, simply find a comfortable posture, preferably with your spine straight, in a comfortable place where you won't be interrupted. Allow your breath to deepen and slow. As you inhale, say your mantra silently to yourself. As you exhale, say it again, silently to yourself. When your mind wanders, gently return your attention to the breath and to your personal word or phrase.

Other Objects of Concentration

You may find that you prefer focusing on something other than a word or phrase. Your object of concentration can be a sound, a fragrance, a love object, or simply an object in nature.

exercise: Practicing with Sound

Sit quietly. Find a comfortable posture, preferably with your spine straight, in a comfortable space where you won't be disturbed. Take several deep, mindful breaths. Close your eyes and bring all your attention to the sounds in your environment, including the sounds that are obvious and the sounds that are subtle. Allow yourself to become totally engrossed in sound without any judgment about what the sound is, what's causing it, or whether or not you like it. Attend to sound fully, just as sound.

The first way that I tried to meditate was by practicing with a simple object. First I focused on a blade of grass until I forgot about other things. Then I tried concentrating on the flame of a candle and later a rose. The idea here, as with all of these practices, is to engage totally in the experience of the object. Whatever the object of your concentration, whenever you meditate, you follow the general instructions of finding a comfortable posture in a space where you won't be disturbed and begin with several deep breaths.

To practice with a fragrance, first you find a fragrance you want to focus on, such as a scented candle, freshly mown grass, or even apple cider warming on the stove. Then, just as you focused on words or sound, you allow yourself to become absorbed in the experience of that fragrance, putting other thoughts and concerns aside when they arise and returning your attention to the sensual experience of smell.

A love object can be anything from your pet to your partner to a spiritual being or symbol. The idea here is to find something or someone you love and intentionally bring your focus to that someone or something. You may do this by visualizing your object of love or by saying its name or by simply feeling yourself in some way close to the love object.

You may want to focus on something in nature that brings you peace. It may be a sunrise or sunset, a beautiful sky full of stars, or the ocean. You can see, feel, and experience nature in your imagination as you meditate, or you can focus on something peaceful and real while seated outside in a natural setting.

Practicing with Numbers

Many people I've worked with find the simple practice of combining diaphragmatic breathing and counting to be the simplest method and the one that's most easily integrated into a busy schedule. Counting backwards from ten to one—with a complete cycle of breath, an inhalation and an exhalation, accounting for a single number—is a simple and effective way to enter meditation.

To practice this way, you start just the way you started mindful breathing in chapter 2. First become aware of your natural breathing. This can be easier if you close your eyes, because that will help you tune out distractions, but closing the eyes is not necessary. To begin, notice where you feel your breath: in your nostrils, in your upper chest, or wherever it is. Now simply let your breath become deeper and fuller until you're breathing deeply enough that your belly begins to move a little with each inhalation and exhalation. With your next inhalation and exhalation, say "ten" to yourself silently. The next time you inhale and exhale say "nine" to yourself. Continue like this until you've finished with "one." You can then open your eyes and return to whatever else you were doing, or you can repeat the counting. Be sure to notice any changes in your stress level. Perhaps you'll find that you're breathing a little more easily, that your body is more relaxed, and that your mind is more focused and peaceful.

You can repeat this many times during a busy day to calm and center yourself quickly, or you can extend it into a longer practice period.

Mindfulness Meditation

In chapter 2, you were introduced to the idea of nonjudgmental acceptance of experience, a core attitude of mindfulness, and to one of its central meditative practices, mindful breathing. You were asked to find a time and place to practice mindful breathing. Take a moment now to review your experience with mindfulness so far. As you do so, remember to practice mindfulness by remaining curious, open, nonjudgmental, and accepting of your experience. Be with what is. Attend to that which needs attention.

exercise: Reviewing Your Experience with Mindfulness Practice

Review your mindfulness experience so far:

1. Have you established a time, a place, and a practice?

   ____

2. If not, what are the obstacles?

   ____

3. What happens when you sit for meditation and follow your breath?

   ____

4. Is there anything you can do to improve your experience?

   ____

5. Are you experiencing benefits from your practice? What are they?

   ____

Whether you've found it easy to practice or you struggle just to stay still for that long, you may be happy to know that mindfulness meditation includes practices other than formal seated meditation. At times when you're more agitated, times when the fertility roller coaster is taking you high and low while rounding a curve, you may find it more difficult to sit for formal meditation. If that's happening, there are other kinds of mindfulness meditations to try.

Mindful Eating

The following exercise focuses your mindful attention on an everyday activity that we usually do without thinking: eating. This trains you to experience deeply and fully an activity of life that we all engage in but don't generally attend to in great detail.

exercise: Mindful Eating

Get a grape and hold it in your hand. Become aware of the weight of the grape in your hand. Hold it lightly and run your fingers over its surface, feeling the smoothness of its skin. Notice its temperature. Perhaps the grape you're holding has been sitting out somewhere and is room temperature. Perhaps it's been in the refrigerator and is cold. Just notice. Place the grape in the center of your palm and let it roll around as you become acutely aware of the sensation in your hand. Look at the grape carefully, noticing the color, the light as it reflects off the grape, and any variations in color or shape. Now hold the grape up to your nose and notice if you smell anything. Touch it to your lips slowly, feeling the sensation of the grape on your mouth. Now, slowly place the grape in your mouth and, without biting it, roll it around in your mouth. Very gradually, put it between your teeth and slowly bite it until you feel its skin break and taste the juice begin to flow into your mouth. When you are ready, but very slowly, begin to chew, allowing yourself to experience all of the sensations of eating the grape. Chew slowly until it's close to liquid and then swallow, feeling and tasting as the grape moves down your throat and into your body.

What was your experience of eating a grape mindfully? How did your experience of the grape differ from your usual experience of eating a grape? Many people, when they first eat mindfully, are amazed at the incredible tastes and textures that are there in the food but go unnoticed or underappreciated in the busyness of a rushed meal. When dealing with infertility, it is extremely important to find pleasure and relief from your fertility focus. Mindful eating can be one way to do just that.

Of course, eating all of your meals at this pace would prevent you from getting anything else done, but hopefully this experience of slowing down and attending to the simple experience of eating a grape has shown you the possibility of increasing the richness of experience simply by giving it focus. You can integrate the experience of mindful eating into your life by eating some meals in silence and allowing yourself to focus on the food and the act of eating it. You can also help yourself to slow down and focus by repeating the mindful eating experience with more grapes or other foods.

Mindful Walking

Mindful walking is similar to mindful eating in that it takes a common daily activity and asks you to attend to it with great focus. This focused attention transforms the activity from a semiconscious routine act into a meditation.

exercise: Mindful Walking

Simply walk, paying attention to all of the sensory experiences of the moment. When thoughts come, and they will, simply let them go, and be in the moment. Do this over and over again.

The thoughts floating through your mind might go something like this: "Blue sky, red rose, am I pregnant? Green grass, weight on feet, cool air, two more days until results. Warm breeze, clouds, children at play, will I have any of my own? Relaxing body, hair in breeze, air in lungs, chest moving, legs stretching, sounds of cars. . . ."

The essence of this practice is to allow your immediate experience to become the meditation. It can be an incredibly relieving experience to simply be in the richness of the moment with all of your senses. This is a really great way to be in nature, meditate, and get some exercise all at once!

A second way to do mindful walking focuses on the sensations of walking. It can be done indoors or out. In this meditation, you simply walk very slowly, feeling the sensation of each foot in great detail as it makes contact with the floor. You can also try coordinating your steps with your breath.

Integrating mindful walking and eating into your regular day-to-day life can help you press the pause button on your fertility concerns and bring you back into the moment. If you're worried about what may or may not happen in the future, you are apt to tune out the present in favor of a feared or hoped-for future. Taking time to eat or walk mindfully can bring you back to the richness of the present moment, the only moment we can really count on.

How to Make Meditation and Mindfulness Part of Your Life

I encourage you to work with all the practices introduced in this book, including both formal seated meditation and the more active practices that you can integrate into your regular activities. Eventually, you will develop some favorites, but first you should experiment and learn what is most helpful to you. You may find that your needs and preferences vary at different times, but your goal should be to establish a central meditation routine that will become a reliable and supportive part of your daily life.

To begin your meditation practice, it's important to make a plan. You're learning a new skill and creating new habits. Establishing your goals and a plan for reaching them will help you find your way and stay on track. You can adjust your plan as you progress, but by having a plan, you will be able to hold yourself accountable and monitor your progress. You might even want to keep a daily calendar with notes about which techniques you practiced, for how long, and with what result.

Creating a Plan and Choosing Your Practices

By now you probably already have one of the most important parts of a plan: a time and place to practice meditation. If not, don't despair. Getting this together is not as easy as it might sound at first. You may need to try several different arrangements until you find something that works well enough to maintain over time. If you're experimenting with different types of meditation and also learning to meditate for longer periods, you may need to adjust when and where you meditate.

Your plan will also include decisions about which practices to try and for how long. Until you settle on a favorite practice or practices, you can review the techniques described in this chapter and begin with whatever practices most appeal to you. You may try using several different practices together and combine the practices that you learned in this chapter with others in the book. For example, you may begin with fifteen minutes of seated mindfulness meditation following the breath, do the counting backwards from ten to one with deep breathing several times during the day, go for a mindfulness walk over the weekend, and eat a couple of lunches a week mindfully in silence.

Developing Support for Your Practice

It's not always easy to maintain your practice. Daily life is always getting in the way. One way to keep practicing is by leaving yourself personal reminders. A reminder can be as simple as a screensaver saying, "Breathe," a note on the refrigerator, or a timer set on your phone to remind you to take a few moments to breathe deeply each hour or two.

Being part of a community all working on meditation can motivate you to keep up your practice. You can join a meditation class or community, or you can practice with a partner. You can even get some virtual support by downloading meditation scripts that can assist you.

Troubleshooting Your Practice

Sometimes when people are beginning to experiment with meditation and challenges arise, they decide they can't do meditation or that it's just not for them. Here are some examples of what can happen:

- Erica fell asleep every time she sat for meditation.
- Lisa couldn't find a good time to practice.
- Jessica's mind raced and she became anxious when she first tried.

Having such problems doesn't mean you will be unable to learn to meditate and reap its benefits. If you encounter a problem, don't give up. Name your problem and try to solve it. Unless you're suffering from severe anxiety or depression, most likely it's a normal part of the process, and you'll be able to solve your problem. Erica, Lisa, and Jessica all solved theirs.

Erica started practicing earlier in the day and using a timer. If she fell asleep sometimes, she accepted it. Eventually her ability to stay awake and yet relaxed increased, and her meditation became a helpful and pleasurable part of her life.

Lisa thought she was too busy to meditate and couldn't settle on a time to practice. When I encouraged her to look more closely at her schedule, she found a lot of wasted time in her day. She concluded that fifteen minutes at the beginning of her day could work for her. After about four weeks of practice, she was delighted to find that, with a clearer mind, she was able to work more efficiently and effectively, and that she actually felt she had more, not less, time for other activities.

After Jessica accepted that it was normal for thoughts to arise, she was able to watch her thoughts without becoming disturbed. As each thought arose, she would say to herself, "Thought," and then return to her breath and the focus of her meditation. Eventually, the thoughts became less frequent and her meditations more peaceful.

As you practice, your experience will change. This is true for everyone. Patient persistence is the key.

Challenge, almost by definition, calls upon us to use resources that we may not look to in calmer moments. As the Chinese character that means both crisis and opportunity reminds us, your response to a challenging situation will vary according to what you bring to it. Developing a strong mind-body practice is one powerful way to survive the emotional roller coaster of infertility.

Key Points

- It's normal to feel you're on an emotional roller coaster when dealing with infertility.
- Understanding yourself and the reasons for your feelings can help you develop more effective coping strategies.
- Meditation is a practice that can help you feel steadier.
- Meditation is a training of the mind that can be beneficial for both mind and body.
- There are two main types of meditation: concentrative meditation and mindfulness.
- You can experiment with different practices and find the ones that work best for you.
- Develop a practice, consider how you can support yourself to practice, and troubleshoot any problems rather than give up. You can do it.

5

connecting to your body

Dealing with infertility can make you feel as if you've lost control of your body. Whether you're worried that you might have fertility issues, you've had problems for a while and are exploring alternative approaches to enhance your fertility, or you've been having difficulty conceiving long enough to be in treatment with a fertility doctor, the bottom line is that your body either is not functioning the way you would like or you're afraid that it won't. If you've experienced repeated frustration and disappointment, you may begin to be angry with your body, feeling that it has betrayed you.

Your body is a major part of your identity. You know how it behaves, how it feels, and what to expect from it. But when you're dealing with infertility, your body may begin to feel alien. If you're in traditional medical treatment, hormones and procedures may make you feel bloated or uncomfortable. Even less invasive approaches, such as dietary changes, changes in exercise, acupuncture, or the use of herbs, force you to be aware of your body in a new and probably less carefree way than before. If you're in treatment, you've surely lost some of your sense of privacy as you've been poked and prodded. To further complicate matters, your intimate life may not be what you would like, since fertility issues are so closely tied with sex and sexuality.

In spite of these challenges, you will want to befriend and work with your body. It may take a conscious decision and some skill, but it is possible. This chapter will show you ways to connect with your body, to nurture it, listen to it, and help it become its most fertile self. First, this chapter will address lifestyle issues, such as diet, exercise, and weight, and review a few practical dos and don'ts related specifically to the care of the body while preparing for pregnancy. An exercise at the end of this section will ask you to explore your lifestyle choices, so you can see how you are caring for your body. This is an opportunity to develop a healthy lifestyle, if you don't have one now, or an opportunity to reinforce good habits and their impact on your fertility, if you do. The Taking Charge section will teach you how to use several mindfulness exercises to elicit the aid of your unconscious to provide a deeper pathway between your mind and your body.

Lifestyle Habits and Your Fertility

There are many things you can do to be sure you're taking care of your body in ways that are conducive to optimal fertility. You may want to pursue some of the issues that will be discussed here with your doctor or with a nutritionist who is knowledgeable about fertility. You may be working with someone such as an acupuncturist or practitioner of Chinese medicine who may have additional beliefs and practices in this area. What follows is a brief review of the basics.

Weight

For many women, weight and body image are a personal and sensitive issue. No one should have to feel that a certain size or shape is superior to another. When trying to give yourself the best chance of becoming pregnant, however, it's important to be neither too heavy nor too thin.

Research indicates that being significantly overweight or underweight can reduce fertility (Al-Hasani and Zohni 2008). The main reason weight is so important to fertility is that estrogen is produced in fat cells. Women who are too thin don't produce enough estrogen, while women who are too heavy produce too much. Many women with either too little body fat and or too much body fat have irregular cycles and don't ovulate adequately or at all. Overweight women also have a higher risk of pregnancy loss. If you are undergoing assisted reproductive technology, being significantly overweight can lower your chances of success (Luke et al. 2011).

To know if your weight is conducive to fertility, you can easily determine your body mass index (BMI); all you need is a calculator and online chart. Your BMI, the relationship between your height and your weight, is highly correlated with body fat. An acceptable BMI for fertility is between 18.5 and 24.9 (Fedorcsák et al. 2004). Of course, the farther you are from the recommended range, the more significant for your fertility. Be aware, though, that BMI is a simple ratio of your height to your weight, and if you're very athletic and muscular, you may have less fat than indicated by your BMI because muscle is heavier than fat.

If you do have a weight issue, the good news is that you can reverse any fertility problems caused by weight simply by gaining or losing it. It's not always easy to gain or lose weight, but if you need to and if you can, it's a wonderful opportunity to take charge of your fertility. If weight management is especially difficult for you, you may want to consider seeking support for this issue. Depending on the cause of your difficulty—whether the issue is physical, or your difficulty relates to emotional over- or undereating, or you need help with selecting healthy foods—you might end up working with a doctor, a psychotherapist, or a nutritionist.

Whatever you think might be the cause of your weight issue, it's always a good idea to start with your doctor to rule out organic problems. If managing your weight is still difficult for you, remember that your weight is only one part of your fertility profile and may not be the one that's causing fertility problems.

Exercise

Exercise is a topic closely allied with weight and one that can have a profound impact on your fertility. Women athletes often lose their menstrual periods altogether, or—even if they do menstruate—may not be ovulating consistently or at all. If you think the intensity of your exercise regimen might be compromising your fertility, you might want to cut back.

Some exercise is always good for your health. Opinions vary on how much exercise is appropriate, so if you're concerned about doing either too much or too little, you may want to check with your own doctor. You also may want to try including gentle exercise, such as walking and yoga, in your routine. It will be a triple win if you do them mindfully: gentle exercise, active meditation, and stress reduction.

Nutrition

Eating properly while trying to conceive is, of course, very important. You want to eat a healthful diet with generous portions of fruits and vegetables and try to avoid processed foods as much as possible. If you're a vegetarian, you need to be sure to get enough protein, because lack of protein can impact reproductive hormones (Barbieri, Domar, and Loughlin 2000). You also will want to consider what kinds of fish you eat, since some are high in mercury, which can harm a baby in utero if and when you do get pregnant. The American Congress of Obstetricians and Gynecologists (ACOG) has specific recommendations on what is safe for you to eat (see resources).

Taking a prenatal vitamin containing 400 mg DHA daily starting at least three months before conception (for both partners) and throughout pregnancy (as opposed to only after you learn you are pregnant) increases chances of conception, and it decreases the risk of several important birth defects (including autism and autism spectrum disorders) by more than 40 percent (Roizen 2011). Just do it.

Herbs

Some people think that herbs, because they're natural, pose no threat and can be taken at random. This is actually not the case. Herbs can have potent effects, and especially when you're trying to conceive, it's important to be vigilant about what you put in your body. It's generally thought that you should avoid certain herbs that can have a deleterious effect on a fetus. Herbs known to be problematic include echinacea, St. John's wort, ginkgo biloba, and blue cohosh (Barbieri, Domar, and Loughlin 2000).

Discuss any herbs that you take with your health care provider to be sure you aren't taking something that could have a negative impact.

Acupuncture

Many women trying to conceive receive acupuncture treatments. Acupuncture has been shown to reduce stress and is thought by many to increase fertility. There have been several studies trying to establish the effectiveness of acupuncture for infertility. One meta-analysis and review of the studies concluded that there is preliminary evidence that acupuncture given before and after embryo transfer improves pregnancy and live birth rates for women undergoing IVF (Manheimer et al. 2008). Researchers continue to explore the impact of acupuncture on fertility.

Tobacco

Tobacco and fertility do not go well together. Tobacco has been shown to be harmful to a woman's ovaries, accelerating the loss of eggs and possibly causing menopause to be reached prematurely. Women who smoke generally take longer than nonsmokers to conceive with IVF and have an increased risk of miscarriage if they do become pregnant. Men who smoke have a lower sperm count and lower motility, as well as increased risk for abnormalities of their sperm. Second-hand smoke is almost as much of a problem. If you're trying to get pregnant, smoking just doesn't make sense (Dechanet et al. 2011).

Alcohol and Caffeine

Even though for many women giving up that occasional glass of wine can be difficult, it's generally recommended that when trying to conceive, women stop drinking altogether and men limit their intake of alcohol. Alcohol can be dangerous for pregnancy and can reduce fertility.

It is suggested that caffeine be limited to no more than 250 milligrams daily, about two cups of coffee (Barbieri 2001). It seems that the combination of alcohol and caffeine is particularly harmful to fertility, because caffeine intensifies the effect of the alcohol (Hakim, Gray, and Zacur 1998).

---

exercise: Exploring Your Lifestyle Choices

Answer the following questions to explore how your lifestyle choices may be affecting your fertility:

1. What is your BMI? Are you inside the recommended range for fertility (18.5 to 24.9)?

____

2. How often do you exercise? What do you do? Do you include light exercise, such as walking and yoga, in your routine?

3. What do you typically eat? Do you eat a lot of fresh fruits and vegetables? Do you eat a lot of processed foods? If you're a vegetarian, what are your sources of protein? Do you ever eat fish that are high in mercury? Are you taking any vitamin supplements?

4. Do you take any herbal supplements? How often? Include herbal teas if you drink them.

5. Are you receiving acupuncture, or have you considered receiving acupuncture to help you conceive?

6. Do you smoke cigarettes? How often? How many cigarettes do you smoke a day?

7. Do you ever drink any wine, beer, or hard alcohol? How often?

____

____

8. How often do you drink coffee or tea?

____

____

9. Are you making healthy lifestyle choices? What area or areas of your lifestyle could you improve upon?

____

____

____

Although it may be a bit of a challenge, adjusting your lifestyle to create a more healthy, fertility-friendly body can lead to a healthier pregnancy, a healthier baby, and a healthier you later on. Try thinking about all the good things you're adding to your life rather than what you're giving up. Imagine you are your own child, for whom you want the best. You are caring for your body gently and with love. You are saying yes to life.

Taking Charge: Working Mindfully with the Body

At this time in your life, when it's likely you're frustrated with your body, finding a way to be present to your body while asking nothing of it can be one of the most valuable things you do for yourself.

In our busy outer-directed world, most people are more focused on the to-do list than on what's going on inside themselves. Even when people are working out, their minds are generally elsewhere as they listen to iPods, watch TV, or think about past or future events. Multitasking is part of our culture and has some advantages, but the downside is that most of us are not present to our bodies until they scream at us in the form of an illness, a headache, or a knotted back. With practice, we can learn to listen to our bodies before they have to scream. Just noticing something as simple as tightness in the shoulders can open the door to an understanding of the presence of tension, as well as to a resolution of the issues, attitudes, beliefs, or fears causing the tension. Our bodies can be a wonderful source of wisdom about our deeper emotional and spiritual selves, if we can just slow down long enough to listen.

This section will introduce you to three different ways to work mindfully with your body: the body scan, progressive muscle relaxation, and autogenics.

The Body Scan

This *body scan* is a wonderful way to begin connecting with the body while making no demands. It's a simple but effective practice in which you check in with your body by bringing your attention to it methodically and mindfully. The best way to do a body scan is without expectation. Simply relax and allow whatever happens to happen. Notice what is, and let it be. You may encounter sensation, thought, or tension. You may feel that nothing is happening, or you may become deeply relaxed. Whatever happens is okay. There is no need to analyze, judge, or run away. It is the truth of the moment, not good or bad. Choose to be with it.

To begin the body scan, find a quiet place where you won't be interrupted. You can read the following instructions to yourself slowly, record them and play them back, or have someone read them to you. The instructions below say to lie down, but if you're sleepy or uncomfortable lying down, it's also okay to sit.

exercise: Doing the Body Scan

Lie down in a comfortable place. If you practice yoga and have a yoga mat, that could be an ideal surface to lie on. Position yourself comfortably on your back with your arms at a slight distance from your sides and your legs slightly apart. If you're uncomfortable, try placing a pillow under your knees or neck. For most people, it's best to lie flat on the floor, but everyone's body is different, and you want to do what's necessary to be able to relax.

Begin by taking some deep, relaxing breaths, allowing yourself to let go of the concerns of the day. You are taking some time now to be with yourself, to be with your body, and to encourage relaxation. Congratulate yourself for taking this time, and allow the concerns of the day to recede.

Let your breath find its own natural rhythm, and begin to focus on the breath mindfully, just as you did in mindful breathing in chapter 2. As you breathe in, you are aware of breathing in. As you breathe out, you are aware of breathing out. Become aware of where you feel the breath. You may feel it most strongly in the nose, the chest, the belly, or the back. You may notice the coolness of the air as it enters your nostrils and the slight warmth as it leaves. Be aware that there is nothing you can do wrong in this exercise. All you're going to do is direct your attention to your body. The mind-body connection will take care of the rest.

And now bring your attention to your left foot. Nothing to do but be aware of your left foot, first the sole of the foot, including the ball of the foot, the arch, the heel, the whole bottom of the left foot. And now bring your attention to the top of the left foot, and to the toes. First the big toe of the left foot, then the second toe, the third toe, the fourth toe, and the little toe. Become aware of the whole left foot before bringing your attention to your left ankle and then your left calf. Feel your left foot, left ankle, and left calf altogether and then bring your attention to your left knee, the front of the knee, the back of the knee, the whole knee. Become aware of the left thigh, the front and the back and now the entire left leg from the bottom of the left foot to the place where the left leg joins the hip. Be aware of the entire left leg.

Now notice your entire left leg, all at once, and compare the feeling in the left leg with the feeling in the right leg. Is it the same or is it different? Bring your attention to the right foot, the sole of the right foot, the ball of the foot, the arch, and the heel. Be aware of the entire bottom of your right foot. Now bring your attention to the toes of the right foot, the big toe, the second toe, the third toe, the fourth toe, and the little toe. Bring your attention to the top of the right foot before moving on to the right ankle, bringing your awareness to the right ankle, the right calf, and all the way up to the right knee, both the front of the knee and the back of the knee. Feel the entire right leg from the sole of the foot to the knee. Now move your attention to the right thigh, front, back, all around the right thigh. Bring your attention to the entire right leg from the sole of the foot to the place where the thigh joins with the hip. And now, bring your attention to both of your legs together, the left and the right, noticing if they now feel the same or if they feel different.

Bring your attention now to your pelvic area, to your buttocks, to your genitals, to your lower abdomen and reproductive organs. Take a breath and simply be aware of your experience as you attend to this area before moving your attention to your low back, your stomach, your chest, your middle and upper back.

Now bring your attention to your shoulder girdle, pausing here to take a few breaths, and then becoming aware of your neck, the place where your neck connects with your shoulders, the whole back of your neck, taking a breath and becoming aware of your whole neck, front and back.

Bring your attention now to your left shoulder, gradually moving your attention all the way down the left arm from the left upper arm through the left elbow, wrist, and left hand. Focus for a moment on the left hand, all of its fingers, the top of the hand as well as the palm. Move now to your right shoulder, your right upper arm, elbow, forearm, and right hand including your fingers and the palm and top of your right hand.

Bring your attention now to your face, your mouth, your jaw joint, the middle of your face, your forehead, and the space between your eyes. Move your awareness to the top of your head.

Now, scan your entire body and bring your attention to any part of your body that calls to you. Allow your entire body to relax and soften. Take your time. As you are ready, begin moving your fingers and toes. You may want to stretch. When you are ready, open your eyes and look around the room until you feel that you are ready to sit up.

Often, it's helpful after an inwardly focused experience to ground that experience in a more outward expression such as writing or drawing.

exercise: Writing about the Body Scan

Take a moment now to write a few words about your experience with the body scan. Writing will help you integrate your experience.

1. What was the body scan like for you overall?

____

____

2. Was any area of your body calling for your attention?

____

____

3. Was any area tense or painful?

____

____

4. How did you respond when you focused on the abdomen and reproductive organs?

____

____

5. Did you feel relaxed?

____

____

6. What did you learn about yourself?

____

____

7. Were you aware of any emotions connected to your body?

____

____

8. How did your body feel after you completed the body scan?

____

____

You can also try drawing your body, highlighting anything that caught your attention during the body scan. You may choose to draw freely or symbolically to express your feelings. Some people enjoy drawing with their nondominant hand to encourage the unconscious to come forth and to alleviate any anxiety about not being an artist. The key is to let whatever happens naturally to occur.

exercise: Drawing about the Body Scan

Use the space provided to draw about your experience with the body scan, or you can use a separate piece of paper.

When you've finished drawing, take a few moments to look at what you've drawn. Notice any emotions that arise as you look at your picture, and complete the following sentences.

Drawing my body was ____

When I look at my body, I feel ______________________________________

My body is ____

My strongest feeling about my body is ________________________________

The word that best describes my body is ______________________________

My overall attitude toward my body is ________________________________

The thing I appreciate most about my body is __________________________

Whatever your feelings toward your body, try to be gentle with yourself and accepting of your experience. Giving attention to your body and to your feelings about your body can bring you valuable information about yourself and help transform any suffering that may exist. Paradoxically, when we come closer to our bodies, listening to them, our bodies begin to soften and our feelings reveal themselves. Our feelings and our bodies are a little bit like children wanting attention. Once we notice and attend to them, they feel comforted and are able to relax.

Progressive Muscle Relaxation and Autogenics

While the body scan is a wonderful, demand-free way to connect to the body, there are times when you will want to encourage your body to achieve a particular end. You can do this with progressive muscle relaxation and autogenics.

Progressive Muscle Relaxation

Progressive muscle relaxation (PMR) is one way to become more active in encouraging your body to relax. As with the body scan, you move your attention systematically to different parts of your body, but with PMR you also tense and release each muscle group. In the body scan you are receptive, whereas in progressive muscle relaxation you are active.

exercise: Using Progressive Muscle Relaxation

Begin by finding a quiet place where you can lie down comfortably. Focus on the breath for a little while, taking some deep, diaphragmatic, relaxing breaths. Bring your attention to your left foot, and tense all the muscles in that foot. Hold the tension for a few seconds, and then relax the left foot completely. Now tense the muscles in the left calf, hold, and let go. Move up now to the left thigh: tense, hold, and relax.

Now bring your awareness to the right foot. Tense, and let go. Let the right foot be soft and relaxed as you bring your attention to your right calf: tense and let go. Now bring your attention to your right thigh. Tense, hold, let the right thigh go limp and relaxed. Now move up to the buttocks. Tense, hold, and let go. Tighten all the muscles in the stomach now. Hold the tight stomach and then let it go soft and relaxed. Continue in this way up through the torso, the shoulders, the neck, and the head and face and down both arms. When you get to each hand, make a fist and then let the hand relax. Scrunch up the face and then let it go soft. End by tensing the entire body and then letting yourself go into a state of soft relaxation.

When you have finished, take some time to relax and notice how you feel. Give yourself a few moments to enjoy and integrate your experience before moving on to the next exercise.

exercise: Exploring Your Reaction to PMR

Answer the following questions to explore your response:

1. How did you feel as you were doing progressive muscle relaxation?

   ____

   ____

2. What did you notice about your body?

   ____

   ____

3. Are you aware of any differences in your mind or body after practicing it?

____

____

4. What did you learn?

____

____

5. Which is easier for you to do: a body scan or progressive muscle relaxation?

____

____

Autogenics

Whereas with progressive muscle relaxation, you were doing something physical to relax your muscles, here you will be working with your mind to make your entire body relax.

Autogenics has an active physical goal but uses an inner process to achieve it. This practice has been used to elicit relaxation and balance in the body since it was first developed in Europe the 1920s. It uses focus, self-suggestion, and mental imagery to encourage the body to produce a parasympathetic, or relaxation, response.

Note that doing autogenics may require a bit of a mental adjustment if you are a very goal-oriented person. That's because autogenics requires that you have a goal (relaxation), but, paradoxically, if you focus too hard on achieving that goal, you will create its opposite: stress. To practice autogenics effectively, you need to follow the procedures and, as much as you can, let go of the results. Autogenics takes practice, so be patient with yourself. Try doing this many times. You'll find that your skill and your enjoyment will increase.

exercise: Practicing Autogenics

Practice autogenics sitting up or lying down in a quiet place where you won't be disturbed. You may like to listen to some soft, relaxing music. Take some deep breaths, allowing yourself to relax. Close your eyes. Now say the following autogenic phrases to yourself, resting after each phrase to allow images to form naturally and easily:

My hands are warm and heavy.
I am at peace.

My feet are warm and heavy.
I am at peace.

My abdomen radiates heat.
I am at peace.

My breath breathes me.
I am at peace.

My forehead is cool.
I am at peace.

My whole body balances itself perfectly.
I am at peace.

What images come to you? For example, when you're saying your hands are warm and heavy, you might imagine yourself warming them near a fire. When you say your forehead is cool, you might imagine a cool washcloth on your forehead. If no images come, it's okay to just say the phrases to yourself. Your mind will still be working on the suggestions. Trust your body to respond.

Repeat each phrase about six times before moving on to the next phrase. After you've gone through the entire set of phrases, repeat the whole sequence again several times.

Autogenics with Biofeedback

I often use a simple do-it-at-home type of biofeedback in conjunction with autogenics. It's not essential, but I suggest that you try it. Several physical changes occur when your body shifts into the relaxation response. Without complex biofeedback and medical tests, you can't measure them all, but one is easy to track. During a relaxed parasympathetic response, the blood vessels dilate, allowing for greater blood flow to the extremities. When this occurs, the hand temperature rises. It's not by accident that "having cold feet" means being worried or afraid of something. With the use of an inexpensive biofeedback device that measures hand temperature, you'll see the immediate results of your practice and be sure that your mind has truly impacted your body.

Using a biofeedback device will also help you perfect your skills by giving you feedback about the effectiveness of how you're practicing. Just as you might be able to guess approximately how much you weigh when your body feels a certain way because you've used a scale in the past, biofeedback can teach you what it feels like to be relaxed.

Biofeedback devices that measure hand temperature come in various forms ranging from little stickers filled with liquid crystal, called *biodots;* to liquid-crystal-filled *stress cards,* which change color like a mood ring in response to hand temperature; to complex biofeedback equipment. I generally use a small, inexpensive stress thermometer that can be found online at biofeedback supply stores (see resources). I prefer it because it has a digital readout that allows you to see temperature changes more precisely than possible with biodots or stress cards, and it costs only about $20.

exercise: Using a Stress Thermometer to Test Your Results

Take your temperature at the beginning and end of your practice. If you decide to use a stress thermometer, tape the end of the device's lead, or wire, to your middle or baby finger as you begin your practice. Use porous tape and be careful not to wrap it so tightly that you constrict blood flow. When you first attach it to your finger, let it register your temperature for two minutes. That's your starting point, your baseline reading. Record it. Then do the practice and look at your temperature again. Most likely it will have risen. If you're able to hold your skin temperature at 93 degrees or above for ten minutes, you have attained mastery, but even a small temperature increase for a short time shows skill and indicates that you're on the right path.

If it happens that your temperature isn't rising, you might be trying too hard, or a medication you're talking might be interfering. Or you might be someone who just naturally has cold hands even when you're not stressed. Once again, let go of results, and if the biofeedback isn't helpful to you, just let it go. You can still practice autogenics. If you do work with a stress thermometer, it's great to keep a log of your temperature readings at the end of practice sessions and watch your skill and your relaxation increase.

With or without biofeedback, autogenics is a great way to relax and reduce your stress. Alternatively, you may find that you prefer one of the other mind-body practices offered in this chapter. Whatever you choose, you will feel better physically and mentally with regular and frequent practice.

Key Points

- Your relationship with your body can suffer during infertility.
- Lifestyle choices can impact your fertility. Treat your body well.
- It's important to connect with your body, to listen to it, and to appreciate it.
- Practice the body scan, progressive muscle relaxation, and autogenics to care for your body and reduce stress.

6

strengthening relationships

Just as your fertility issues create stress for you, they can also create stress in your relationships. They can impact your relationships with your husband or partner, your friends, your family, your colleagues, and even your casual acquaintances. As you focus on your fertility, some relationships that worked well in the past may become strained, while others may deepen. It's possible that some friendships may drop into the background for a while as new friendships develop in response to your changing needs and interests. This is a time to become conscious of who is in your life and whether they support you or drain your energy. It's a time to let go of any unnecessary shoulds, to set limits with others where appropriate, and to surround yourself with loving friends and family.

In this chapter, you will read about some of the common relationship issues and dilemmas faced by women dealing with fertility issues. As you read, consider your own relationships. Some exercises will help you explore and evaluate your current relationship life and how your fertility issues affect it. You'll be asked to tune in to your feelings and your needs. There will be guidance in managing difficult emotions and difficult situations. The Taking Charge section will offer exercises to help you identify, accept, and communicate your desires. It will emphasize ways to strengthen your bond with your partner. The important thing at this time is that you open yourself to an honest evaluation of your feelings and needs so you can be your own best friend and advocate.

Exploring Your Relationships

Relationships that are especially pleasurable or especially problematic tend to catch our attention, but we have many relationships that affect us in more subtle ways. It can be helpful to explore your entire relationship life. A great way to begin your exploration is to create a relationship map that includes all the people you're in contact with, beginning with the most intimate and central and extending to those you see as part of your life but whom you know only slightly.

exercise: Creating Your Relationship Map

In the space below or on separate paper, draw five concentric circles, or circles inside other circles. You'll need to make them large enough to be able to write in. In the center, the smallest circle, write the name of your husband or anyone else who is intimate and at the center of your life. In the next circle, write the names of significant family members and, in the next, the names of friends. Moving outward to the next circle, write the names of people you know through your work, and in the last circle the names of those you know most casually. Here you might want to include people whose names you might not even know, such as a friendly person who works in your office building or a familiar salesperson, as well as people you see in your neighborhood, church, gym, or elsewhere but don't know well. As you work with this map, be aware that you can't do this wrong and there will be some people who could be named in more than one circle.

After you've completed your map, take a few moments to look at it mindfully. Think of it as a kind of aerial view of your relationship life. Reflect on what it felt like to create it and how it feels to look at it. Circle the names of the people who bring the most light into your life and underline those who create issues for you, drain your energy, or deplete your spirits. Are there any changes in your relationship life that you would like to make? Include changes that you would like to make even if you don't think you can make them. How much time do you spend with people who uplift you? How much time with those who create tension or drain you? Can you increase your contact with the positive people in your life? Write your thoughts in the lines below. Is there an action plan you can adopt?

____

____

____

____

____

____

____

____

As you worked with your relationship map, you may have noticed particular kinds of issues, in specific circles or categories. For example, you may have noticed the most conflict in the family circle and the most support in the friendship circle, or you may have noticed just the opposite.

Different types of relationships may present different issues. Here are some common issues by relationship category. See if any fit for you.

Friends

Women in general are nurtured by their relationships with others and, in times of stress, often are comforted by something as simple as a good conversation. It can be particularly difficult if, while stressed with fertility-related concerns, there are any conflicts or ambiguities in relationships that have been supportive in the past. Even a good, solid friendship can become stressed while dealing with fertility.

Friends often are unaware of what it feels like to deal with fertility problems and may, without realizing it, say or do hurtful things. If this happens, you may not know how to respond. It may seem that you have to endure the emotional upsets or give up on your friendship. On the other hand, your friend may do nothing insensitive, but if she is pregnant or has children, you may be uncomfortable with your own feelings of envy or anger or sadness when around her. Like many women I've known, you may find yourself increasingly avoiding people and situations that include pregnancies and babies or, if not actually avoiding them, wishing you could. It can be very distressing to find that you are unable to be comfortable with someone whose love and support have been important in your life. You may value the friendship but feel it slipping away as your circumstances and your friend's circumstances diverge.

Family

The issues with families are similar to the issues with friends but—depending on your family dynamics—can be even more intense. While you may choose to skip a party at someone's house, you may not want to miss Thanksgiving or avoid a niece's first birthday. Issues with our mothers can be very intense at any time. Whatever your relationship with your mother, it's apt to become more pronounced at this time. Your mother may be a great support to you, but on the other hand, her anxiety for you may feel like a burden, her concerned questions may seem intrusive, or her advice might miss the mark. Mothers generally mean well when they tell their daughters to relax, or to adopt, or to enjoy the freedom of childfree living, but it's not what you want to hear when you're doing everything you can to become a mother, just as she already is.

One of the more difficult family situations is when a younger sister has children and you don't. Some women feel that without children, they're treated differently from brothers and sisters who are already parents. You may feel that people are tiptoeing around you, afraid to mention pregnancies or births for fear of upsetting you or, conversely, that people talk at length about children and pregnancies. This is a situation in which you may not be sure of what you want. It can be uncomfortable to feel people are treating you differently, and it can also be painful to hear about others becoming parents. Feelings of sadness, envy, or anger may arise from time to time even if your overall feelings about your family are loving and positive.

The Office

People often say that you can choose your friends but not your family. While this is true, it is nonetheless possible with both friends and family to make some choices about whom you spend your time with and when. In the case of coworkers, this isn't always the case. You have to pass the pregnant receptionist every day or be in a meeting with others who are talking about their children. You also generally have less freedom at work to discuss your needs and feelings. If you're out of the office frequently for medical, fertility-related reasons, you may wonder whom—if anyone—you should confide in about your situation.

Casual Relationships

Casual relationships—people you see in your daily activities or acquaintances who aren't central to your life—can nonetheless impact your mood and your sense of well-being. Whether it's the teller at the bank who asks you how many children you have, the building service worker who hands out cigars on the birth of his child, the friends of friends who meet you for lunch and ask questions about the fertility process—all of these interactions can be upsetting. In fact, many people may ask you if you have children, and precisely because you don't know them well, you find it difficult to know how to respond.

Your Partner

Your relationship with your husband or partner will, of course, be affected by fertility issues. You may both have strong feelings about what's going on, but your individual reactions and needs may differ. If you and your partner have different ways of dealing with emotional issues or conflicting ideas about how to handle issues, you may feel suddenly more alone than before. It's common to blame a partner who wasn't ready to start a family earlier, when you may have been more fertile. Sometimes one person wants to pursue treatment longer and try more options than the other does. And one partner might want to adopt or use donors or surrogates, while the other doesn't. In any of these situations, home life can be pretty challenging.

There can also be issues if your emotional styles or needs aren't working harmoniously. I have often found that women want to be listened to and have their feelings validated, while men tend to want to fix things. The fix-it approach can feel unempathic to you if it's not what you need, and your husband will suffer feelings of helplessness since he can't fix the problem. Of course, this gender split is not perfectly consistent—some men want a sympathetic ear and some women want to take charge—and regardless of gender, people deal with problems differently. Nevertheless, if one of you wants to talk about problems and the other likes to avoid them and focus on other things, it can be difficult to find a comfortable balance. And it can be incredibly painful when the infertile spouse fears the other will abandon the marriage to seek a fertile partner elsewhere. I've never seen this actually happen, but I have heard many women express such a fear.

exercise: Evaluating and Improving Your Relationships

Take some time now to think of specific people and situations in your life that sound similar to the ones you've been reading about. Focus on your relationships in each category. Answer the questions below to guide your through this process. Try to be honest with yourself about your feelings. Remember, most people have a mixture of positive and negative feelings and experiences, even about people they love the most. Write about what works well in your relationships and about what doesn't.

1. Have any of your relationships changed since you began having a fertility focus?

2. Which relationships are most supportive?

3. Which relationships have issues?

4. Would you like to see less of someone or more of someone else? If so, who are they?

5. What makes you feel good in specific relationships?

6. What situations or circumstance have made a relationship difficult?

7. Are there certain relationship issues that make you feel helpless or trapped? What are they?

____

____

8. What changes can you make to get the love and support you want from the people who know how to give it?

____

____

Managing Strong Emotions in Relationships

The emotional stress of infertility can cloud your perception of yourself and others, making it difficult to manage relationships in ways that are in your own best interest. If you're feeling very emotional, you may judge or mistrust your own reactions. You may not understand your feelings clearly or know when your needs are legitimate. You may want to talk to others about your reactions but wonder whether doing so would be appropriate. If you're feeling broken or inadequate in any way, you may be afraid that others will judge you or feel sorry for you if they know how you feel. When you're feeling emotional, you may not be sure of where the line is between your emotions, the situations you encounter, and the behavior of others.

It's important to remember that what you're feeling is not unusual. In all probability, the situations and comments that bother you would also bother most women with fertility issues.

Natalie's Story

Natalie, a woman who attended my mind-body fertility group, was quite emotional as she went through fertility treatments. She recognized that she wasn't the optimistic, outgoing, and generous self she used to be, and she felt uncomfortable with who she thought she had become.

Natalie was particularly distressed while taking the fertility hormone Clomid. When her best friend talked incessantly about her wonderful pregnancy and the pleasure she had from her first child, Natalie couldn't stop crying. She felt embarrassed by her lack of emotional control and began to distrust her reactions. Because she questioned the appropriateness of her feelings, Natalie also questioned her right to tell her friend that she preferred not to hear about the life events that were making her friend so happy. She was hurt and angry but felt that she should continue her friendship without saying anything.

When Natalie joined our mind-body fertility group, she began to realize that certain comments and situations, including having a friend talk at length about the joys of motherhood, are almost universally disturbing to women with fertility challenges. Knowing that others felt as she did didn't remove the upset Natalie experienced, but it did help her trust and validate her own emotional reactions. It also made her feel less alone and gave her the confidence to make clearer decisions about how to handle the situation. When things got uncomfortable with her friend, Natalie could envision herself telling the story to the women in her mind-body group and would feel relieved and better able to cope.

Natalie began keeping a list of situations that had disturbed her. Here's her list:

- *Baby showers*
- *Pregnant women at work*
- *Pregnant siblings*
- *In springtime, seeing so many women expecting*
- *Stores full of young children*
- *Holidays, especially Mother's Day and Father's Day*
- *My mother talking to her friends about my fertility challenges*
- *People asking for details about my treatment, including asking me about results*
- *Others acting so upset that I begin to feel I'm burdening them*
- *People minimizing and acting like I'm making a big issue out of nothing*

Natalie also made a list of comments that she hated to hear:

- *"How many children do you have?"*
- *"What are you waiting for?"*
- *"Why don't you just adopt?"*
- *"My friend adopted and then got pregnant right away."*
- *"You're just too stressed out. Relax!"*
- *"Why are you so emotional?"*
- *"We would like you to take charge of the office baby showers."*
- *"What are you buying Shauna for her new baby?"*

- *"Thanksgiving will be at your sister's this year so we can see our grandchildren."*
- *"When are you going to make us grandparents?"*
- *"You're not getting any younger."*
- *"You'll really be sorry later if you continue living your selfish childfree life."*

Making these lists helped Natalie maintain perspective and trust her feelings. Sometimes she could even laugh a little about it.

Do Natalie's lists remind you of reactions you've had to similar situations and comments? In the following exercise, you can write down situations and comments that have bothered you.

exercise: Recording Situations and Comments That Disturb You

List the situations and comments that you've found troublesome:

____

____

____

____

____

When other situations arise that disturb you, remember that what you're experiencing is what many women have experienced. You can stop second-guessing your emotions.

Please take comfort in knowing that you are not alone. Of course, how you choose to handle similar comments and situations will have a lot to do with the specifics of the situation and your own personality. However, the next section offers some guidelines for managing your relationships while managing fertility.

How to Improve Your Relationships

Now that you've explored your relationships and how they're affecting you, here are some tips for how to think through your relationship issues, choose which relationships to concentrate on, and feel more comfortable with the people in your life.

Validate Your Feelings

It is important to accept your feelings. This doesn't mean you have to love having those particular feelings. It means only that you recognize that they are there legitimately, for good reasons. You are okay, and your feelings are also okay even when they're uncomfortable for you. You may be like many women who long for a baby and beat themselves up emotionally when fear, anger, sadness, and envy make it hard to be totally happy at the news of a friend's pregnancy. These feelings are normal, though painful. If you're starving, it's hard to rejoice at the feasting of others. You can be gracious to your pregnant friend, but you don't need to fault yourself if you can't fully share in her happiness.

Figure Out What You Want

Even those who love you the most can't read your mind or intuitively know just what you want. Many people who know what you're going through don't know how to act around you when the subject of babies comes up. Even you may not know what you want from others. Try to figure out what you want. Do you want to hear about family members' new babies? Do you want to hear about your friends' kids? Before you can ask anything of others, you need to know what you'd like to ask.

Decide Which Relationships to Focus on Right Now

Use your relationship map to help you focus your energy on the people who are important to you now and in the future. Commit to the important relationships in your life even if they take work. Spend as much time as possible with people who make you feel good. Minimize contact with people who add stress to your life. Like Natalie, develop new friendships with others who share your experience with fertility issues. It's much easier to share your feelings with people who are going through what you're going through.

Communicate Your Needs to Others

Of course, you won't tell everything to everyone, but on the other hand, it's fine to ask the people who know and care about you to avoid difficult subjects when around you.

When you want to request a change in someone's behavior, always begin with the word "I" and then describe your feelings. Generally, people are doing the best they can and will become defensive if they feel attacked or criticized. You want to communicate in a way that accomplishes your goal without creating hard feelings. Saying something like "When you talk to me about your pregnancy, I feel uncomfortable" will be received differently from telling someone that they're being insensitive and hurtful to you by talking about their pregnancy.

Avoid Unnecessary Misery

There are some people whom you will want to educate about your needs and others whom you will want to avoid as much as possible. Give yourself permission to avoid situations and events that are too distressing. If you think you should be happy for someone who's having a baby shower but know you'll be absolutely miserable if you attend, consider staying away. If it's a very close friend, you may even be able to discuss your feelings honestly and ask if she would mind terribly if you skipped the party. You may be able to say no more often than you realize.

Be Realistic about What You Can Change

A random person probably will ask you how many children you have, or someone in your office will announce that she's pregnant. Unaware comments and the pregnancies of others can be painful reminders of your struggle but are generally not intended to hurt you. Some women spend a great deal of energy being angry with others for asking a question that was intended as a friendly gesture. When a random person asks you a question in an effort to show interest in you, a simple answer such as "None yet, but we're hoping for children in the future," followed by a quick change of subject, can sometimes be the best course. And when the subject is unavoidable, you can work within yourself to remain as calm and optimistic as possible.

Take Care of Yourself

This is a time to be your own best friend. Soothe, balance, and pamper yourself. Practice the mind-body techniques that you've learned. Work with your thoughts, write in your journal, be mindful, breathe, and meditate. Know and accept your darker feelings and then invoke the positive—positive images, positive feelings, positive people, and positive situations. There will be resolution. This is not your entire life; it is just a time in your life.

Taking Charge: Knowing and Communicating Your Feelings

Having good relationships at any time involves knowing and communicating needs and feelings while respecting the needs and feelings of others. Even if you've done this effectively all of your life, the challenges of infertility can bring you into unfamiliar territory. The practices in this section will help you know your feelings, tame the ones that are difficult, and communicate with the people in your life who are most important to you.

Knowing Your Feelings

Eugene Gendlin, a psychologist teaching at the University of Chicago in the 1970s, studied therapy outcomes in order to learn what made some therapy clients more successful than others in meeting their therapeutic goals. His observations led him to identify a specific skill set used spontaneously by the successful clients, which he was then able to refine and codify into a remarkably effective therapeutic system called *experiential focusing*, which is used to this day. In his book *Focusing*, Gendlin (1981) identified specific steps for focusing on feelings to understand them deeply.

As you deal with fertility, you will encounter feelings and situations that are new to you. I've found that using a simplified version of Gendlin's systematic way of attending to your feelings can deepen your understanding of your reactions.

exercise: Experiential Focusing

Find a quiet spot where you can sit undisturbed. Take a few mindful breaths and allow yourself to settle into the present moment.

Now ask yourself a question about a feeling you've been having. As you do, pay close attention to your body. What do you feel? If you're not sure, try naming your feeling with different words, such as "anxious," "fearful," "sad," "wistful," "nostalgic," to see if any strike a chord.

If you notice something happening in your body in response to your question, delve deeper by asking yourself what it's about. Wait quietly for an answer to come to you. You will know the answer is correct when you feel a subtle shift in your body.

Continue in this way, asking each new thought, feeling, or sensation what it's about, and going deeper and deeper.

Experiential focusing can be both subtle and powerful. It may take a while to learn, but when you practice it effectively, it will reveal your deeper feelings and needs. Whatever you find, accept it and honor it.

Kim's Story

Kim thought she knew all about her reactions to her mother, but by using experiential focusing, she learned even more about herself and was able to make positive changes in this important relationship.

Since first encountering fertility issues, Kim had been upset with her mother, who seemed to always know how to say exactly the wrong thing. When Kim told me about some of her mother's upsetting comments, it became clear that although her mother occasionally said something insensitive, she was doing her best to support her daughter. She was saying things that weren't always exactly on target and could be annoying, but she wasn't saying anything that, on the surface, should have caused such extreme distress. Kim decided to use experiential focusing on this difficult issue.

Kim began by taking a comfortable position and tuning in to her body. She asked herself, silently, what the issue with her mother was all about. Had she not been focusing in a specific way, she might have talked to herself about how insensitive all of her mother's remarks always were, but because she was using the focusing technique, she simply asked the question, attended to the sensations in her body, and waited. As she did this, she noticed a tightening in her chest, a kind of ache. Delving deeper, she asked herself, "What is this ache?" She tried different words and listened. Her first word was "sad." When she said, "Sad," she felt a subtle shift in the sensation in her chest. Then she heard the word "heartbreak." She experimented with the words "angry," "jealous," and "resentful" and felt subtle shifts with each, but the big shift came when the word "lonely" floated up.

When she asked herself about the loneliness, an underlying issue began to unfold. Kim had always been very close to her mother and considered her a role model for her own future, which she'd always thought would include having children. In the past, Kim was always able to identify with her mother and felt sure that her mother understood her well enough, but when it came to the possibility of not being able to conceive a child, her mother seemed really clueless. She had never experienced what Kim was experiencing now. She had had children easily. Kim felt a separation from her mother that she had not felt before. It was frightening and upsetting. It almost felt as if her mother had turned on her. Kim felt deeply alone.

Kim left the session ready to talk to her mother. Instead of withdrawing and feeling like an angry victim, she was able to express both her love for her mother and how she would like to be treated while dealing with fertility. She bridged the gap between them by explaining her experience more clearly and helping her mother understand how to be helpful to her. Kim continued spending time with her mother, who became one her greatest supports. Instead of letting her fertility concerns rob her of an important relationship, she had let them be the impetus to deeper communication and a closer bond.

Focusing is a technique you can practice whenever there's an issue or feeling you want to understand more fully. If you find some feelings difficult to tolerate, give yourself permission to do this exercise only insofar as it feels safe and productive. If you discover feelings that you want to reject because you think you shouldn't have them or because you're ashamed of them, remember that such feelings as anger, resentment, and envy are experienced by most women dealing with fertility problems. These feelings don't mean that you're bad in any way. Accept your feelings as messages to yourself. Knowing yourself more deeply may not only make you feel better but also provide a road map for making your relationships better.

exercise: Creating a Focusing Log

Since you won't always have time to focus deeply when a difficult situation occurs, you can use the following space to log some of the issues, feelings, or events you want to focus on. Then make a date with yourself to use focusing at a point when you'll have more time. You also can use this log to record anything of note from earlier focusing sessions.

Date/Time to Focus	Issues, Feelings, or Events to Focus On	Focusing Notes

Taming Difficult Feelings

If you're feeling emotionally overwhelmed, your strong feelings will affect your relationships. And sometimes you'll want to be able to tame those feelings as well as understand them. You may be able to use focusing alone to tame your feelings, since focusing, in addition to providing insight, often causes feelings to become less intense. But you may also want to consider two other techniques described in this section: pillow talk and meridian tapping. As you learn these new skills, remember to continue practicing the breathing, meditation, and imagery skills you already know. You can always return to the safe-place imagery that you learned in chapter 1 if your feelings become too intense.

Pillow Talk

When dealing with fertility issues, it can be as though you've placed a small bucket outside during a very heavy rain. If your emotional bucket gets too full, it may begin to spill over in ways that aren't good for you or your relationships. Before that happens, you can choose to empty it. At times, you may be able to share your feelings in all their intensity with someone very close. As long as you don't direct your feelings at that person and you have an agreement that it's okay for you to share feelings in this way, an intense emotional expression, especially when followed with a hug, can bring you closer to the other person.

There may be other times, however, when you're looking for ways to empty your emotional bucket on your own, either before talking to someone about an issue or just to feel better. *Pillow talk* is a way of doing that. Instead of talking to a person, you talk to a pillow, allowing yourself to express all your anger and sadness. If you're angry with a particular person, you can yell at the pillow. If you're angry with infertility, you can pretend the pillow is infertility. You can't hurt the pillow with your feelings. You can yell at it and hit it. If anger isn't the feeling you're trying to express, you can simply talk to the pillow. I promise it won't talk back, so you'll be able to express your feelings without interruption, and that alone can be calming. You may find afterwards that you're able to speak more calmly with the people in your life and take better care of your relationships.

If this exercise is working well, you should feel some relief when you've finished. If you find that it intensifies your feelings and you don't feel relieved after a little while, it might not be the best approach for you. If that's the case, don't worry. There are many other approaches in this book to work with, and all are designed to help you balance your emotions. Honor your own preferences.

Meridian Tapping

Meridian tapping is a term that covers several tapping therapies, including thought field therapy and emotional freedom technique (EFT) among others. These therapies have developed in recent years, and although they are still considered experimental, I've found them very helpful in my practice.

Meridian tapping is based on the idea that the body has an energy system. If you've ever tried acupuncture, you're most likely familiar with the concept of *chi*, or energy, and energy *meridians*, or pathways. Meridian tapping is sometimes called emotional acupuncture, because it's done by bringing a thought, emotion, or sensation into awareness and then tapping on a series of acupuncture points. The goal of meridian tapping is to balance the energy and thereby reduce or eliminate the distress associated with unpleasant beliefs or experiences. Meridian tapping reduces stress and is also thought to balance the body.

The idea that we all have an energy system and that we can work with that system directly to achieve greater well-being has been part of traditional Chinese medicine for thousands of years, but it has not been a part of Western medicine. Depending on your beliefs and experience, it may seem strange to you. Even if you do feel comfortable with the concept of energy meridians, you may find it strange to tap on your body. I suggest that you give the technique a serious try. It's simple to do, and I've seen it be very effective. One of the great things about meridian tapping is that you don't need to believe in it for it to work. In fact, when I introduce it to people in my office, they often find it strange or unbelievable but still get good results. It's presented here as a way to reduce difficult emotions, but you can try it on anything physical or emotional. It's even possible that it can help clear stress-related obstacles to fertility.

To practice meridian tapping, you will want to find a comfortable space where you won't be disturbed. This technique can be practiced in any position. You will want to read through all of the instructions in the next exercise before you begin working on an issue. You can use the Meridian Tapping Points diagram to find your tapping points.

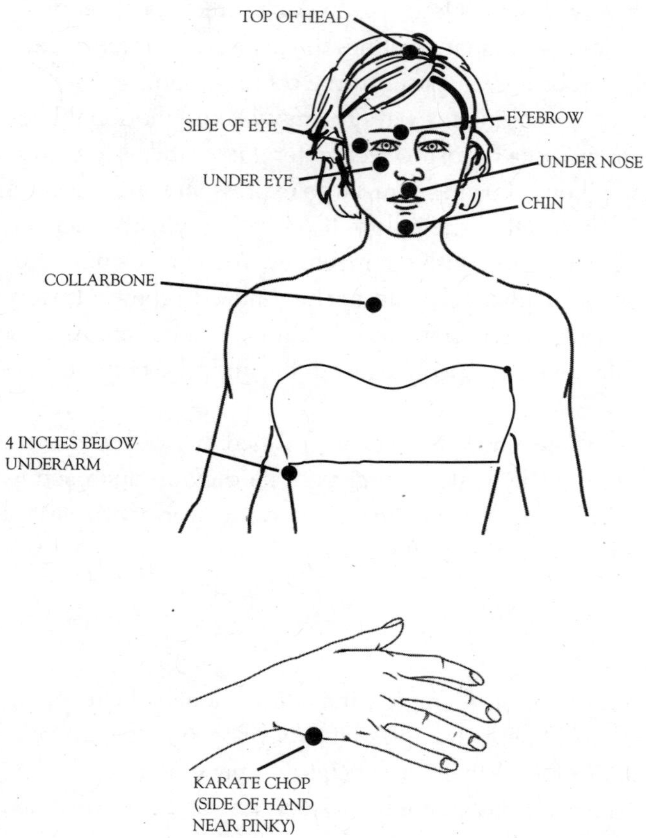

Meridian Tapping Points

exercise: Practicing Meridian Tapping

Identify an issue that's causing you distress. It can be any emotion or situation that makes you feel uncomfortable. Call the issue by name—for example, "discomfort around my mother."

Attend to the feelings in your body that accompany the issue, and very subjectively rate your distress level on a scale of 1 to 10, with 10 being the highest and 1 the lowest level of distress. This is your starting point, your baseline. As you're learning this technique, you may want to begin by working with issues that you would rate between 5 and 7 on the scale. Later you can take on more challenging emotions. The idea is that tapping will reduce your distress, and your distress level—or number—will go down.

Next do the first part of the tapping sequence, called the *setup*. Use four fingers and tap gently on the karate point on the side of your hand (see diagram).

As you tap your hand, say aloud the following sentence, inserting your own issue: "Even though I ______________, I deeply and completely love and accept myself." Insert "feel discomfort around my mother" or "am angry with my friend" or whatever issue you've identified. Repeat the phrase three times while tapping. Paradoxically, acceptance clears the way for change. This is an important part of the process, so even if it seems strange or difficult, be sure to start with the setup.

Next, move on to the second part of the process. Use two or three fingers and tap on the rest of the highlighted points in the diagram while saying the name of the issue out loud. You can start at the eyebrow point and end with the top of the head, as I do, but the exact order of tapping points is unimportant. There is also no need to worry about whether or not you're tapping on the exact spot. You're tapping on a point where an acupuncture needle would go, and since your fingers are so much larger, you can't miss. There is no set number of times you have to tap, but something like seven is typical. No need to count.

- Tapping on the eyebrow point, say your issue (for example, "angry with my friend Sarah").
- Tapping on the side-of-eye point, say your issue.
- Tapping on the under-eye point, say your issue.
- Tapping on the under-nose point, say your issue.
- Tapping on the chin point, say your issue.
- Tapping on the collarbone point, say your issue.
- Tapping on the below-the-underarm point, say your issue.
- Tapping on the top-of-head point, say your issue.

Now repeat the entire sequence. Notice if your body starts to relax a little. Think about the issue and rate your distress level again on a scale of 1 to 10. Is the number the same as when you first rated your distress, or has it gone down? Occasionally, as you tune in to your issue, you'll feel it more acutely for a while, so the number will go up temporarily. If this happens, continue tapping. Eventually, you should find some relief or change.

If you notice movement to a new emotion or a new aspect of the same issue, it's a sign of progress. You can tap on this new aspect. For example, you may reduce your anger but find you're feeling sad. You can then tap on the sadness.

After you have tapped on the unpleasant feelings and reduced your level of distress, you may also choose to tap on the same points but using words such as "I feel calm and accepting" that express how you would like to feel. This tapping can help you continue to reduce the intensity of your emotion and move toward inner calm.

Meridian tapping, along with pillow talk and experiential focusing, can help you manage the strong emotions that accompany fertility issues. Doing so will help you in all of your relationships, including your relationship with your partner.

Communicating with Your Partner

Your partner in your quest for a child no doubt shares in your disappointment when news is discouraging, but despite your common goal, your experiences with fertility and his won't be exactly the same. If the road to parenthood has become rocky, you will want to be able to connect across the differences in order to remain supportive, compassionate, and close. Many couples have told me that fertility problems have created marital problems but say that facing this challenge together has made them stronger as a couple.

This section is here to give you guidance and skills to help you strengthen your bond now and in the future. Good verbal communication will help you stay connected to your partner. This section will teach you two useful communication techniques: temperature reading and active listening. It also will address obstacles you may encounter in your sex life as you're dealing with fertility issues, and suggest ways to overcome them.

Taking a Temperature Reading

When dealing with fertility stress, the time pressure created by multiple appointments, and the all-too-frequent presence of unpleasant emotions, it's easy to avoid talking, to hit dead ends when you try, or to have an inordinate amount of your conversation focused on fertility. When feelings are intense or conflicted, people often think communication means discussing problems when, in fact, it can mean sharing, connecting, staying in touch.

Taking a structured *temperature reading* can help you stay connected and keep your communication balanced. Years ago, a family therapist named Virginia Satir developed such an exercise. A temperature reading isn't intended to take a long time, nor is it a way to solve problems. It's a check-in comprising a series of statements and questions that you and your partner share with each other. One of you asks and listens without commentary or argument, and then the two of you exchange roles. It's a form of structured conversation that asks you to address the entire range of your experience and then share it with your partner.

Frequently, couples find this style of communication awkward and stilted when they first try it but later come to value it highly. I hope you'll try it and stick with it. It's best to do this while sitting face to face, holding hands, and making eye contact, but sometimes couples aren't able to do that and choose to communicate by phone, text, or e-mail. Remember that when you are the listener, your job is to listen. It's okay to repeat or briefly summarize what the speaker has said, but asking questions or inserting your own opinions or issues will disrupt the process and make it less safe. With a little time, you'll smooth out any wrinkles and develop your own, more natural style.

exercise: Taking Your Temperature Reading

Use a coin toss or other random method to decide who is to speak first while the other listens. Then do the following as a couple to help you stay connected:

The first speaker makes a statement of appreciation. Here's a chance to focus on things that you value about your partner but may not always mention. Your appreciations to your spouse may be about something you have always valued about him or something he just did. For example, you might say something like "I appreciate the way you always stay steady and focused" or "I really appreciate your cooking dinner last night." The only requirement is that what you say is something you honestly feel good about.

Next, the first speaker shares some inside information. This information should be something going on for you that your partner might like to know. It may be an internal stress that could potentially influence mood and behavior, or it could be some news that would be good to share.

The first speaker then poses a question. This should be something you don't understand or you're wondering about: "Did you get the tickets for the concert?" "What made you so late last night?" "Are we still on for dinner with your family next week?" "How are you feeling now about this fertility process?"

The first speaker then lodges a complaint and asks for a change. This part of the check-in can help you express specific complaints while requesting specific behaviors that would make you happier. This is important, since often we have complaints about something but either can't formulate a positive alternative or can't communicate our needs in explicit and understandable ways. Remember, however, that this is just a check-in designed to help you stay in touch on a variety of subjects and not a time to engage in long problem-solving sessions on difficult topics. If a difficult issue arises, you may want to agree to discuss it later with active listening, which is another technique you'll learn in this chapter. For the temperature reading, you will want to keep it fairly contained and specific. Ask for something that your partner will understand and be able to do, not something that asks him or her to have a different personality.

The first speaker then offers a hope for the future. Refocusing on your hopes and dreams as individuals and as a couple can provide the perfect ending to your check-in, one that allows you to reconnect with your future. One of your hopes, of course, will be to have a baby, but you should also offer other hopes. Hopes can also be short term, such as "I hope we can take some time together this weekend that's just for us."

After completing the cycle, the first speaker thanks the listener for listening. Then the second speaker has a turn and takes the same steps: offering an appreciation, sharing some inside information, posing a question, lodging a complaint and asking for a change, and offering a hope or dream.

Structured temperature readings can help you balance a focus on fertility with the rest of your relationship, as you may choose to discuss fertility, other issues, or both. You may want to have some temperature readings that are open to any topic and others that focus on only one topic, such as fertility. The temperature reading can be a contained way to share information about your medical input, treatment options, and emotions.

Here is how two couples—Tina and Steve and Marlene and Sam—used their temperature readings.

Tina and Steve's Fertility-Focused Temperature Reading

Tina and Steve's temperature reading was focused on fertility issues. Tina spoke first:

Appreciation: *"I really appreciated your coming home on short notice when I told you I was ovulating. I also appreciated your making dinner when you saw I was upset."*

Inside information: *"I'm hoping that I won't have to move forward with fertility treatment. This is the last month we agreed we would try on our own. I'm hopeful but scared."*

Question: *"I'm wondering if you know your travel schedule for work and if you'll be here when I find out whether or not I'm pregnant."*

Complaint with request for change: *"I find it upsetting when you don't let me know about your travel schedule until the last moment. I would really appreciate your sending me an e-mail or talking to me directly as soon as you get your schedule so I can be prepared. I know it can change later, but then just let me know if it changes."*

Hopes and dreams: *"My hopes and dreams are obvious. I hope I get pregnant this cycle. I'm anxious to move on into pregnancy and parenthood. My overall dream is for a happy family life with you and our children."*

Steve spoke second. Here's what he said:

Appreciation: *"I really appreciate you for trying so hard to do everything possible to encourage pregnancy. You've changed your diet, you've given up wine, and you're practicing meditation, all so that we can be parents."*

Inside information: *"I have a lot of stress at work right now. They're making some structural changes in the company, and I want to position myself correctly. I know I can be short-tempered sometimes, and I want you to know I'm sorry for that. It's not about you, and I want to do better."*

Question: *"I'm wondering if you've decided which doctor you want to see if you're pregnant and who you would want to see if you're not. Will you want me to go to an appointment with you?"*

Complaint with request for change: *"I know you really want a baby and are always thinking about that. I know you want to talk about it, but I really want us to talk about other things, as well, and put some fun back in our lives. I would really appreciate it if we could put some time limits around how much we discuss fertility, maybe fifteen or twenty minutes, and then go on to other things."*

Hopes and dreams: *"I share your dreams of a family. We have so much love to share. I hope it will happen soon."*

As mentioned, you can use structured temperature readings to cover general topics. The following reading between Marlene and Sam is a good example of how this can work.

Marlene and Sam's General-Topic Temperature Reading

Sam was the first to speak:

Appreciation: *"I appreciate the way you encourage me in my work. It means a lot to me."*

Inside information: *"As you know, I've been working out. I'm really happy right now because I've reached a new fitness level, and I feel quite a bit less stressed after working out."*

Question: *"I'm wondering if you're still going out with your friends this weekend, or if we could get tickets for a show."*

Complaint with request for change: *"In the morning, your alarm is going off repeatedly and waking me. I understand that you need the alarm to get up, but I would appreciate it if you could try to organize yourself so you don't have to snooze the alarm so much."*

Hopes and dreams: *"I really love you and our marriage. I'm dreaming of the time when we're in a new house with a new family. That will make it even better."*

Marlene spoke second.

Appreciation: *"I really appreciated your making dinner for us last night. It was great!"*

Inside information: *"I just learned that I'm being considered for a promotion at work. I'm pretty stressed about it. On the one hand, it would be great for my career, but on the other hand, I'm not sure I would want to have such a demanding job at this particular time. You said that I seemed preoccupied. It's not about you. I'm just thinking about my work situation more than usual."*

Question: *"I'm wondering if you were able to order the sink for our new bathroom and if you've talked to a plumber about installing it. Is there anything I need to do now to help complete the project?"*

Complaint with request for change: *"When you work out until eight o'clock every night, we aren't able to have dinner together early enough for me. I'm getting up earlier in the morning now, and I would like to go to bed earlier. I would love it if you could find a different time to work out, at least for part of the week."*

Hopes and dreams: *"You know I'm always hoping to be pregnant. That's number one, right now. I also am dreaming of living near the water and having a boat. Of course, the biggest dream is for a long and happy life with you."*

Avoiding Common Pitfalls During Temperature Readings

Taking a daily temperature reading is one of the most valuable couples exercises I know, and I hope your experience with this technique is a good one. But if you're having difficulty with it, here are some troubleshooting tips.

When you disagree: Sometimes it's hard to listen to what the other person is saying without arguing. Your perspectives about situations may be different, but when this happens, take a deep breath. Remember, you're learning more about what your partner is thinking, which can help you resolve differences in the future. You will never agree on everything. It's how you handle disagreements that will make the difference between a happy marriage and a stressful one.

When you feel impatient: Sometimes it's hard to sit back and listen when you feel like you have so much to say, too. This is another time to take a deep breath. There will be plenty of time later to be heard. Right now, you're validating your partner by listening.

When you have difficult emotions: It can be really difficult to listen to another person and contain your own emotions, especially when that person is complaining or asking you to change. With couples, it's easy to react with strong emotion because you are important to each other and the emotional stakes are high. But it's for this very reason that you're doing this very structured exercise. Trust your ability to resolve issues, and focus on what is good, positive, and strong in your relationship.

Mad, Sad, Scared, and Glad Check-In

One variation of the couples check-in is called Mad, Sad, Scared, Glad. You can use it as part of a general or specific temperature reading when you're revealing inside information. It also can be used by itself as a way to check in with your partner. It is especially helpful when you have a lot of tension or agitation and don't know exactly what you feel. It's another tool for calming emotion, because getting clear and even talking about how you're feeling usually reduces the emotional energy. Here's an example of one woman's Mad, Sad, Scared, and Glad check-in:

Mad: "I'm angry that this process drags on so long. I'm annoyed that I'm the one who has to do most of the procedures and deal with the doctors. I'm angry that having a child had to be this difficult for us. I wanted it to be easier and fun. I'm angry that my mother asks me every day about how it's going with the 'baby thing' even though I told her it was uncomfortable to talk about it so much and to let me bring it up."

Sad: "I'm sad that having a baby can't be more fun and enjoyable. I'm sad that you get left out of a lot of the process so much when I know you care too. Sometimes I despair that after all this struggle, it won't work out. I miss the ease of our relationship and am sad that so much time is taken up with fertility."

Scared: "When I feel apart from you, I get scared that this will drive us apart. Sometimes I worry that you feel like I'm failing or not doing enough. I'm afraid we won't be successful. I'm scared that you will get impatient and want to stop trying before I do. I'm afraid life will never feel normal again."

Glad: "I'm so glad you want a baby and are willing to go through this with me. I'm so grateful for the kindness of the doctor and his staff. I'm glad I have a mom who wants to support me and will be such a good grandma. I'm glad I have such good health habits. I'm pleased with myself for all the new things I'm learning and doing, like meditation and focusing, that will be good for me, no matter what."

As this example illustrated, you start the check-in with mad, move through sad and scared, and finish with glad. You can cycle back to any of these emotions if you need to, but be sure to thoroughly explore each one before ending. This is also a good tool to use with journaling or writing. It is a way to allow your emotions to move and not stay trapped inside.

Active Listening

During the temperature readings or at other times, issues and feelings may arise that need more attention. The next exercise will show you how to use *active listening* to give a structure for talking about issues at greater length. Some version of this practice is recommended by most schools of couples therapy. It offers both of you a way of saying what you need to say without interruption or retort and a way to listen deeply.

Most of the time when people are conversing, the listener is busy formulating a reply even before the speaker has finished. This is especially true if the topic being discussed is emotional or controversial in any way. In active listening, the listener concentrates instead on listening closely to the speaker and validating the speaker's feelings by reflecting them back in words. As you practice active listening, you and your partner will be able to express yourselves fully and know that you've been seen and understood. It can be an amazing feeling and can bring you closer.

As in the temperature reading, active listening offers each of you the opportunity to speak and be listened to in turn. Again, you begin by choosing who will speak and who will listen. Later, you will switch roles and have an opportunity to be heard.

Practicing Active Listening

Sit across from each other, looking into each other's eyes and holding hands. Decide who will speak first and who will listen. Then take the following steps to listen actively to each other:

1. The speaker expresses his or her own thoughts and feelings, pausing after short segments. For example, in an active listening session between Tina and Steve, Tina might say: "I find it upsetting when you don't let me know about your travel schedule until the last moment. I would really appreciate your sending me an e-mail or talking to me directly as soon as you get your schedule so I can be prepared. I know it can change later, but then just let me know if it changes."

2. The listener responds to the speaker by reflecting the essence of what she or he has heard, and then checks to be sure he or she hasn't misunderstood or missed something. As listener, it may be difficult at times to withhold reactions and comments, but being able to do so is essential to making this practice effective. As an example, Steve might say to Tina: "I hear you are saying that you want me to communicate with you about my travel schedule as soon as I have it. Have I understood you, or did I miss anything?"

3. The speaker either corrects the listener's understanding or acknowledges it and continues. Tina might say: "Well, yes, I want you to communicate with me, and I also want you to understand that your schedule affects me. When I don't know what to expect, I can't make plans that work for me. I spend a lot of time at home alone, when I might have made other arrangements if I'd known earlier that you would be out of town. I don't really like spending so much time alone right now, because I have more of a tendency to worry when I'm alone."

4. When the speaker is done, the listener makes a statement beginning with words like "Given all that, it makes sense that. . . ." The listener then validates the speaker's feelings with a sentence or two that shows understanding. Steve might say: "Given all that, it makes sense that you would want to hear from me sooner so that you can plan your time when I'm away. You may want to see friends or go to a yoga class or have a massage, or something else, but since I don't generally let you know when I'll be out of town until the last minute, you can't make arrangements and are left with nothing planned."

5. The speaker thanks the listener for listening. In addition to a simple thank you, a wonderful way to appreciate your partner for listening is with a hug.

6. The speaker and listener then change roles and repeat each of the active listening steps, so that the former listener now has a chance to be heard.

Just as with the temperature reading, this practice can feel stilted in the beginning but will bring great rewards if you give it a chance. Sometimes just slowing down and hearing each other can work miracles.

After each of you has had a turn being both speaker and listener, you may want to contemplate your experience. Here are some things to consider and, perhaps, discuss.

- How did it feel to be the speaker and to be listened to?
- What was it like to be the listener?
- Do you feel different in any way as a result?
- Is there anything you understand about your partner now that you didn't understand before?
- Can you name a way in which you feel better understood than before?
- As you think of yourselves as a couple, what is different as a result of doing this exercise?

Integrating Skills to Make a Marriage Stronger

While each of the relationship skills has been introduced in this chapter as a separate practice, you can use them in an integrated way, according to your needs. The following story shows how Nicole used them in her relationship with her husband, Adam.

Nicole's Story

Nicole was feeling uneasy in her relationship with Adam when she was going through fertility treatments. She used experiential focusing on her feelings about her husband and realized that their difficulty discussing their fertility issues was driving them apart. They had a great relationship overall, but not being able to discuss important issues was like having a giant gorilla in the room that no one dared acknowledge. Their relationship was growing increasingly distant. Nicole was feeling lonely and wanted to feel closer to her husband.

Nicole and Adam began practicing daily temperature readings, which brought them closer and helped them to bring the fertility topic into their conversations more often. Nicole was pleased with the progress she was making in connecting more closely with her husband, but she was often left with fertility-related questions and requests for change that were just dropped. Nicole realized that some of the issues that arose during the temperature readings needed more attention.

She made a list of those issues and made dates with her husband to address them using active listening. Here is a small part of their first active listening dialogue and a summary of the solutions they ultimately reached.

Nicole: *I really feel lonely. I go to the doctor alone most of the time. I know you also want a baby, but I'm the one who has to go through all the procedures. I feel afraid to talk about my feelings to you because I'm thinking that you just hate it when I cry, and you don't know what to do. When you tell me to "relax, it will be okay," I feel cut off and lonely. I don't want you to be uncomfortable, but I wish we could find a way to talk more.*

Adam (actively listening and reflecting): *I hear that you're feeling afraid to talk with me about your feelings in relation to fertility. You go through all the procedures and feel you can't talk to me as much as you would like. You feel cut off when I reassure you. Am I understanding everything you are trying to tell me? Is there anything I missed or misunderstood?*

Nicole: You have most of it right. I also want you to understand how very lonely I feel.

Adam: Given what you have told me, it makes sense that you would be feeling very lonely. You take the brunt of all the appointments and treatments and then feel uncomfortable sharing your feelings with me because of my response. I see how alone that must make you feel.

Nicole went on to explain her experiences in more detail while her husband reflected. When she felt she had expressed what she needed to express, they switched roles. Her husband explained how helpless he felt when he saw her upset and how uncomfortable he was with not being able to make things better. He liked feeling in control, and the unpredictability related to fertility made him anxious. Nicole was able to hear him and reflect his meaning. Understanding each other made them feel closer.

Ultimately, Nicole and Adam were able to work out a plan that was comfortable for both. Nicole explained her needs to be listened to and allowed to express herself. She explained that, for her, knowing that she could share feelings with him was all she wanted. He felt relieved knowing he wasn't expected to find a solution. Respecting the fact that he felt uncomfortable with long emotional sessions, they agreed to set some boundaries around how much time they spent focused on the fertility issue and to keep the conversation about their respective needs open.

Are any of Nicole's issues similar to yours? Do you have feelings or issues that you would like to communicate more fully, whether they're about fertility or some other topic? You may want to make a note of any issues you're aware of and make a date with your partner to address them with active listening. Here are some fertility-related questions that the two of you may want to consider:

- Are you communicating well enough regarding factual matters, such as medical findings and treatment options?
- Do you find that you are both in agreement most of the time when it comes to decision-making related to fertility?
- Are you able to discuss feelings easily? Is this true for both of you, or does one of you feel the need to hold back? If so, why?
- If you do express your feelings, do you feel happy with the response you receive? If not, what would you like to be different? Have you communicated this with each other?
- Do you agree about how much you want to discuss fertility? If not, what would you each like?
- Have you discussed how you feel about sharing your fertility information with others? Are you in agreement about what you should tell and with whom you will share this information? How do you decide what to do if you're not in agreement?
- Have you discussed how long you will try to conceive, and have you considered other options? If so, are you in agreement?
- Does either of you blame the other or feel that you're letting the other down?
- Are you marking turning points in your fertility journey together with ritual, celebration, or just a time to be together? Does what you're doing now work for both of you?
- Are you replenishing and nurturing your relationship with pleasurable activities?

exercise: Making a Date for Active Listening

Come up with a list of issues that you want to discuss with your partner and make a date to address them through active listening. You and your partner can each add to this list or make separate lists.

Date/time for active listening ____

List of topics to discuss ____

____

____

____

____

General Principles of Good Communication

Sometimes couples fear bringing up topics that may be contentious. Research on the strength of marital relationships has shown that strong couples don't have any fewer areas of disagreement or conflict than couples with severe problems. The difference comes in how they treat each other and how well they connect (Gottman and Silver 2000). Following these basic principles of good communication can help keep you close, even when differences arise:

- Be respectful. Scorn, contempt, blaming, and name-calling can drive you apart.
- Own your feelings. Ask yourself who has the problem. Begin your sentences with the word "I" to avoid blame.
- If you have something to criticize, begin with something positive. Say something positive first. Then let the other person know specifically what you would like to be different. Name how making this change might benefit the other person and the relationship.
- Stick to the topic at hand. It can be tempting to load on, but not helpful.
- Learn to share and learn to listen. Keep a balance between the sharing and listening.
- Don't expect an immediate solution. Some things are unknown or have no easy fix, but communicating will keep you close as you experience ups and downs together.
- Communicate your needs. Some people assume their partner will or should know what they want. Take responsibility for saying what you need.

Frequently couples are doing their best to show their love and concern for each other but are missing the mark. The tendency to expect our partners to read our minds can cause hurt feelings and anger. To remedy this, you can each make a list of what makes you feel loved. Before doing the next exercise, you can photocopy it for your partner.

exercise: Making Your List of What Makes You Feel Loved

Sit quietly with yourself and think of ten things that make you feel loved. Be specific. For example, saying "I feel loved when you show interest in me" leaves room for confusion and misunderstanding. Saying "When you approach me to do a temperature reading, I feel cared about" or "I love it when you spontaneously kiss me" will give your partner the information he needs to make you happy. It's okay to ask.

Use the following space to list what makes you feel loved:

1. ______________________________

2. ______________________________

3. ______________________________

4. ______________________________

5. ______________________________

6. ______________________________

7. ______________________________

8. ______________________________

9. ______________________________

10. ______________________________

After your partner makes his list, you can share your lists.

When your partner does something from your list, you should acknowledge and appreciate it. He should do the same for you. You can add to your lists over time. Some people keep their lists on the refrigerator as reminders.

Improving Your Physical Relationship

Infertility or suspected infertility will impact your sexual relationship. This is true whether you're trying to get pregnant with your partner in the bedroom or with the help of your fertility doctor. By acknowledging issues and communicating with your partner, you don't have to allow this important aspect of your marriage to be damaged. Your sex life might be a little different for a while, but it's possible that in the long run you will be able to make it even better than before.

The problem is that infertility affects your sex life by tying your sexuality to the task of conceiving. Spontaneity and passion can go out the window, and sex can become an obligation or demand tied to your ovulation cycle. If your possible pregnancy is now in the hands of a doctor and a lab, sex can remind you that you were not able to produce a child through your lovemaking. If you've been through a lot of treatment, your relationship to your own body may have temporarily been disturbed, making it more difficult for you to feel sexual. But there are things you can do to keep your sex life fun and rewarding. Here are a few of them.

Communicate. Share your feelings about your sexual relationship, how it might have changed, and any thoughts you have for making it better.

Experiment. This is a time when the old tried-and-true might need to change. Open yourself to variety. Share fantasies. Don't be afraid to play.

Accept. Accept that some things might be different for a while, but also know that this time can be an opportunity to become closer.

Affirm. Infertility doesn't make a woman less of a woman or a man less of a man, but it can often feel that way. Affirm yourself and your partner. Remember, the brain is a major sexual organ.

Cuddle. Stay close physically even when not being sexual. Just cuddling can feel fabulous and strengthen your emotional connection.

The bottom line for you as a couple trying to have a child is that your desire for a child together grows from the bond you already have. Right now you're facing a challenge together. Contrary to what most of us think, sharing the vulnerable feelings that arise during this time creates an opportunity for deeper intimacy and bonding. Sharing the joys and sorrows of the experience and learning new ways to connect and communicate your feelings and needs can bring the two of you closer than either of you ever imagined, now and in the future.

Key Points

- Fertility stress can change relationships.
- It's helpful to review relationships as a whole and emphasize the positive.
- The origins of strong feelings can be elusive during infertility.
- Use experiential focusing, pillow talk, and meridian tapping to understand and rebalance intense emotions.
- Communicate and share with your partner. Temperature readings and active listening are helpful methods of doing this.
- Staying physically close to your partner can help you stay emotionally close.

7

resolution

Regardless of the way in which it occurs, at some point the fertility struggle itself comes to an end. You become pregnant on your own or with the help of assisted reproductive technology. You decide to adopt, or you choose to live without children. Whatever the resolution for you, it involves letting go of what came before, with all of its hopes, dreams, and struggles, and it involves embracing the outcome, with all its new possibilities for satisfaction and joy.

Trying to become pregnant when it doesn't come easily requires focus, commitment, and determination. Every time you are disappointed and then choose to try again, you affirm the importance of bringing a baby into your life. You expend more and more capital—emotional, physical, social, and financial—because you so badly want to catch that gold ring, your biological child. Even when you catch that gold ring and find yourself pregnant, it may take a little while for you to feel secure enough in your pregnancy that you can begin to prepare for being a parent. And if pregnancy doesn't come, and you decide to let go and do something different, it's not always easy to adjust to a new dream.

This chapter will help you understand the issues involved in adjusting to different possible outcomes. It will give you some new tools to help you assess your options if you are trying to choose whether to continue with treatment or to move on. The Taking Charge section reviews all the mind-body tools introduced in this book and how they can help you as you move from one stage of your life into the next.

Pregnancy After Infertility

Getting pregnant after a struggle with infertility or suspected infertility is joyous. It is what everyone wants, the overwhelming first choice. But a period of infertility leaves an emotional trace that surprises many couples even as they celebrate a pregnancy. This is something you will be able to manage better if you are aware of the issues.

Adjusting to pregnancy after infertility involves changing teams, so to speak. In the past, you may have looked at pregnant women as the ones who couldn't understand what you were going through. You may have been angry with them or envious of their good fortune. You may even have tried to avoid them. Now that you're pregnant, you're one of them, but you feel a little different because pregnancy was something you had to work for. You probably have friends who are still where you were so recently, still trying to get pregnant. You may suspect that they're not feeling so friendly toward you now that you're on the other side. And you may have old friends whom you avoided during your fertility struggle, and now you're wondering how to rekindle those connections. You are adjusting to a new social reality.

If you've struggled to become pregnant, you may also be nervous about maintaining your pregnancy, not because there is any medical reason to support this fear but because it feels a little unreal and impossible that everything is finally working out as you would like. You've been hopeful and then disappointed so many times in the past that it's hard to trust either your good fortune or your body. It may seem odd to go to the obstetrician and be just another pregnant woman. You may wonder why you can't be monitored more closely, even when closer monitoring is unnecessary, or you may be especially cautious about testing during pregnancy. You may need to wait until you've worked through some of these issues to openly allow yourself to celebrate with others.

The following exercise will help you begin to reorient to a sense of yourself as a parent-to-be.

exercise: Using Mindfulness to Shift from Pregnancy to Parenting

Find a quiet place where you won't be interrupted. Breathe mindfully, allowing your body and mind to soften and relax. Approach your experience with open acceptance.

Allow an image to form of yourself pregnant. Notice the many changes large and subtle that are happening to your body. Notice how you feel about the child that is now developing in your body.

Breathing deeply, allow any feelings you have to arise and move through your attention— fear, joy, gratitude, anger, sadness, pleasure. Allow yourself to see the pregnancy progressing through the various stages and finally arriving at the birth of your child. Who is present for this birth? Notice and allow the feelings that arise.

Allow an image to form of yourself as a parent. Notice what presents itself first. What do you see when you think of yourself as a parent? Take your time, allowing yourself to be aware of your experience. Notice what your child does and how you respond. Play with your child. Hold your child. Teach and love your child. Watch him sleep and wake up.

Be aware of what you enjoy about parenting and what fills your heart. Be aware that once you are a parent, you will continue to be a parent as long as you are alive.

Keep breathing and imaging yourself as a parent, trusting that as you do this, you will become more and more settled into this new way of being that your developing child brings for you.

As your pregnancy continues, you will grow more confident and comfortable. Gradually, the struggle with fertility will recede as your life becomes filled with the joys of parenting.

Moving On without a Biological Child

It can be really painful to let go of the dream of having a biological child. With the rapid development of reproductive technologies today, you have treatment options that didn't exist a few years ago. Each treatment option has a cost and a possible reward. This is true of medical interventions and even some alternative treatments you might be exploring. You may not be clear about how far you should go and at what cost. If things don't seem to be working out, you may not be sure about when to let go and move on. Here are a few things you will want to consider.

Consider the costs. Compare the cost of what you're doing with your emotional, physical, and financial reserves. You may decide you want to try eight IVFs, use donor egg or sperm, or, if medically appropriate, use a surrogate. On the other hand, you may want to save your money and your energy for adoption, or you may want to change your focus and let go of trying for a child, at least for a while. You will have some guidance for some of this from your medical team, but many choices will be very personal and not always clear-cut. You and your partner may have to look deeply within for answers.

Revisit your reasoning. Why did you begin trying to have children? Evaluate the importance of each reason from your current perspective. You may feel strongly about passing along your genetics or about experiencing pregnancy and birth, so if you can't do that, you may prefer to live childfree. On the other hand, the most important thing for you might be the experience of parenting, and you may feel ready to go out and find your child through adoption.

Imagine possible futures. As you've been trying to have a biological child, it may have seemed that there was only one way for you to be happy. You may have thought more about yourself with a baby than as the parent of a school-age child or adolescent. Imagine the possibility of happiness with other outcomes and at different stages of family life.

exercise: Why Do You Want to Be a Parent?

Think about the reasons you want to be a parent. List the reasons here. There's no right or wrong, better or worse. This is to help you listen to your own heart.

____

____

____

____

____

____

The part of becoming a parent that was important to you when you began trying to become pregnant may have changed. Listen to yourself as you are now.

Deciding What to Do Next

If this is a time when you're making decisions about what to do next, stepping back from the intensity of the moment and seeing where you've been can help you evaluate your options. Creating a timeline of your experience from the time you decided to have a child until now can give you perspective.

exercise: Creating Your Fertility Timeline

On a large piece of paper, draw a long horizontal line. This line represents the period of time that you've been trying to become pregnant. On the left end of the line, write the approximate date you decided to try to become pregnant. At the opposite end of the line, on the right, write today's date. Fill in the key moments in your journey from then until now. Include your whole experience—the time of trying on your own, the worry, the decision to see a fertility specialist, the tests, the procedures, the major decisions, and the results.

As you think about your timeline and consider where you are right now, what are your strongest thoughts and feelings about your experience so far? Do you know what you would like to do next? What really stands out for you as you look at your timeline? Write your thoughts in the space provided.

____

____

____

____

____

Having considered your fertility journey from the beginning to the present moment, you will be better able to assess your options moving forward.

Deciding when to let go and move on is a very personal decision. If you do decide to move on, you will have to grieve the loss of your dream of having a biological child, but if parenthood is what you're after, you most likely still have options.

exercise: Weighing Your Options

Consider the future, including all the options and the pros and cons of each. Make a list of your choices as they are right now. Include any choices you have for continued treatment. If you're considering other options, such as adoption or childfree living, list them.

Next to each choice, write down the pros and cons. Consider the impact of each option on your emotional resources, your body, your finances, and your relationship life. Look at how your life might change if you choose to let go of treatment. Ask yourself what's most important to you right now.

Options	Pros	Cons

You and your husband or your partner can make separate lists and then share them with each other as you decide on your next steps. If your priorities are not exactly the same, try using some of the skills you learned in chapter 6 to move your discussion forward in a spirit of harmony and respect.

Deciding to Leave Treatment

It can be very difficult to make the decision to leave treatment if you're offered any hope of success and if having a pregnancy of your own is very important to you. The following story shows how one couple made a decision with the help of the exercises presented in this chapter. This couple's timeline, option review, and final decision may be similar to yours or totally different. That's unimportant. You have your own story, but seeing how Megan and Rob worked through their situation may give you some new ideas about your own.

Megan and Rob

Megan and Rob, a couple I worked with in therapy, struggled to become pregnant and had difficulty deciding when to let go of treatment. Megan had tried to become pregnant for three years. Each time anyone offered any hope or possible treatment, she chose more treatment. When her original reproductive endocrinologist told her it was unlikely she could conceive using her own eggs, Megan chose to try using donor eggs. She did conceive during two donor cycles but lost both pregnancies.

Thinking perhaps a different doctor and a different protocol might help, Megan traveled to a clinic that offered a new approach and new hope. Again, she conceived and lost the pregnancy. She was devastated. She cried all the time and could barely function at work.

Rob tried to cheer her up, but this led Megan to think he just didn't understand how tough it was for her, which left her feeling more desperate and alone. The new reproductive endocrinologist was prepared to try another cycle with a new protocol that she thought would give Megan a better chance, but this time Megan wasn't sure she wanted to go on. She was exhausted and heartbroken.

To help them decide what they wanted to do next, Megan and Rob made a fertility timeline of all they had been through related to fertility. They drew a long line on a large piece of paper. As they recorded the significant steps along their fertility journey, they remembered how things had been. They remembered the worry that had developed as they were disappointed month after month. They remembered when their ob-gyn suggested that they see a fertility specialist and have a workup. They remembered the early testing followed by IUIs, the medications that made Megan depressed, the injections, the endless doctor visits, and the nervous waiting for results after procedures. Sadly, they remembered all the heartbreaks and how each time they had regrouped to try again, because they so desperately wanted a baby and there still was hope.

As they worked on their timeline, they were aware that they were still candidates for more treatment, if they decided that's what they wanted. They had been told it could be worth another try. After all they had invested, they didn't want to give up. Maybe the next cycle would be the time they would succeed and their dreams would come true. On the other hand, they were tired. Extended fertility treatment and multiple losses had taken a big toll. They wanted to pull back and assess the costs and possible benefits of various options.

Writing down their options and considering how they felt about each helped them look at their situation more objectively. Here's what Megan and Rob's list of options looked like, with the pros and cons they associated with each possibility.

1. *Another donor egg cycle*

   Pro: *I will feel like I have done everything possible. There's a chance it will work, and then everything will have been worthwhile. I feel sad we can't use my own eggs, but this gives me a chance of having a baby with some characteristics of my husband.*

   Con: *I most likely will be disappointed, and I'm not sure I can handle more loss or more hormonal upheaval. It's expensive. The investment of time, money, and emotional energy keeps me from pursuing other goals like travel and career. I'm worried that we're putting ourselves in a financial situation that will make it difficult to adopt if that's what we decide to do. I'm sick of the stress and of doctor visits.*

2. *Surrogacy*

Pro: *We could have an infant with Rob's genes.*

Con: *It's so expensive it would put us in a difficult situation.*

3. *Moving On*

Pro: *We put the struggle behind us and do something we know will make us parents.*

Pro: *We're not totally attached to passing on genes, but we are totally attached to being parents. If we stop treatment now, we can pursue adoption while we're still young. We can even take the vacation we've been talking about to renew ourselves and our relationship. I can get my body back, and we can get our lives back.*

Con: *It's really hard to let go of something we've wanted so badly. As long as I stay in treatment, I feel there is some hope, even if it's small.*

4. *Adoption*

Pro: *We will definitely become parents. We'll be able to do fun things with our children and share our love. We will have equal relationships with our child, since the child won't be biologically connected to either one of us.*

Con: *As a couple, we won't have a biological connection to our child. It's not what we had hoped, and we will have to grieve the loss of having our own biological child. It may be more difficult, though not impossible, to get an infant.*

When they really focused, Megan and Rob realized that some of their goals and priorities had changed over the past three years. Many of their friends now had children, and the reality of diapers and crying babies was not as attractive as they had initially imagined, but they really did enjoy the older children in their lives. Megan had put her law career on the back burner while trying to become pregnant, and having watched her colleagues move ahead, she was anxious to put more energy into her career. She and Rob had put the purchase of a new home on hold and had never taken that trip to Hawaii they had both dreamed of. They were aware that they were growing older and that this could be their time to enjoy some things that might be more difficult to do once they were parents. Now that they had clarified their needs and priorities, Megan and Rob were ready to make a decision.

Megan and Rob decided to discontinue treatment, give themselves time to adjust, and then adopt. They took the trip to Hawaii that they'd put on hold, and they bought a new house. Megan had more energy for her legal career. And they now have a beautiful adopted daughter whom they adore. Whatever sadness they may still carry from their years on the fertility roller coaster—and their inability to build their family in the way they had initially hoped—it is overshadowed by the joy of the family they now have. While in the midst of treatment and uncertainty, they never would have believed it possible.

Choosing Adoption

If you arrive at the decision to adopt, you will need to allow yourself some time to grieve the loss of your hopes for a biological child before you can open your heart to the child you will parent. You will also need to make some decisions about how you would like to move forward with adoption. You may choose to work with an agency as you pursue domestic or foreign adoption. You may also want to look into private adoption. Each state and each program has its own laws and requirements, so you will want to educate yourself about adoption in your area.

After Megan and Rob decided to leave treatment and pursue adoption, they, like many couples who make this decision, felt sad to be giving up on a biological child but were relieved as well.

As Megan and Rob noted to me, if you choose to adopt, you are no longer wondering whether you will become a parent. The question, instead, becomes when and how it will happen and who your child will be.

Deciding to Live Childfree

Sometimes when people run out of options for further fertility treatment or decide they would no longer like to pursue treatment, they also decide they would rather not adopt. Sarah and Adam were one such couple.

Sarah and Adam

Sarah and Adam had dreamed of being parents from early in their relationship. They loved thinking about how their children would look. They imagined a composite of their best characteristics. When they learned that they had fertility issues, they were scared their dream would not come true. They tried everything they could to have a child, but at some point they ran out of treatment options. Their choices were adoption or childfree living.

Sarah and Adam considered their priorities and their options. They imagined themselves as parents of an adopted child. They listened to their hearts. After much contemplation and discussion, Sarah and Adam realized that they were not interested in adoption. They were motivated to create a child together but not to parent a child who was not biologically their own. They were wise enough to know themselves well and to respect their own preferences.

Sarah and Adam reassessed their lives. They both had challenging and exciting careers that involved a fair amount of travel. They had a great relationship and enjoyed each other. The day Sarah announced that she and her husband had decided to remain a family of two, she seemed almost as happy as other women have been when telling me they were pregnant. She had resolved her fertility issue in the best way possible and was relieved that the struggle was over. She had accepted the outcome and could see a life ahead that, although not the life she had imagined, would be nonetheless meaningful and happy.

Some couples, like Sarah and Adam, decide the best thing for them is to find new dreams and to point their lives in a different direction. It's not an easy decision, and not everyone embraces it as Sarah did. If you're considering childfree living, you will need to grieve what didn't happen and look to the future. You may focus on interests and goals that were pushed to the side while you tried to become pregnant. You may refocus on career, hobbies, travel, or saving for a fabulous retirement. Free of the struggle for children, you may find new pleasure in your relationship with your husband or partner.

While you're in the midst of trying to create your family, it may seem impossible to find happiness without children, but many couples have gone on to prove otherwise. There may be more than one path to fulfillment for you if you open yourself to new possibilities.

Times of Transition

If this is a time when you are transitioning to parenthood or childfree living, it's also a time to take stock of where you've been and how far you've come. Sometimes in life we feel we're climbing a mountain. We only look up and fail to look back to see all the progress we've made. Even when things don't work out just as we wished, we have still moved forward by doing what we needed to do to be true to ourselves. When something is left behind in the past, there is more room for a future to form and to be embraced.

Taking Charge: Living Mindfully

Whatever your outcome, all the mind-body practices introduced in this book are still there to enrich your life. Meditation, mindfulness, journaling, imagery, and working with thoughts and emotions all are practices for a lifetime. However you use them and in whatever context, they can be vehicles for a more fulfilled life. Here's a quick reminder of the skills you've learned.

Diaphragmatic breathing. Breathe deeply, allowing the breath to fill your lungs. Your belly will rise slightly as you do this. With this one simple technique, you're on your way to relaxation. (See chapter 1.)

Imagery. Create an image of yourself in a safe place for stress relief and emotional balance. Experience yourself as strong and solid as a mountain, whenever you want to feel stable or when you need perspective. (See chapter 1.)

Cognitive behavioral therapy. Work with your thoughts. Be aware of your mental habits and create realistic optimism. (See chapter 2.)

Mindfulness. Mindfulness is an attitude and a practice. Be in the moment. Follow the breath. Meditate. You can do anything mindfully, including walking, eating, doing the dishes, caring for a child, anything. (See chapters 2 and 4.)

Concentrative meditation. You can meditate by focusing on one thing. Choose something that brings you joy and peace as the object of focus. It can be the breath, a word, a feeling, or an object. There are many choices. (See chapter 4.)

Journaling. Writing down your thoughts, feelings, and memories can help you be healthier and happier. There are many ways to journal. You can release your emotions, organize your thoughts, have a space for creative expression, or remember to be grateful. It's your choice, so do it your own way. (See chapter 3.)

Connect with and care for your body. Listening to your body with the body scan can help you tune in to yourself while releasing tension. You can use progressive muscle relaxation and autogenics to relax and find balance. (See chapter 5.)

Care for your relationships. Knowing your needs, releasing and tempering your feelings, and communicating effectively can bring you the joy of connection. The temperature reading; active listening; mad, sad, scared, glad; and physical closeness will strengthen your relationship with your partner. (See chapter 6.)

Care for yourself. Practicing experiential focusing, pillow talk, and meridian tapping will help you connect with yourself, release strong emotions, and reduce distress. (See chapter 6.)

Key Points

Life is a journey. We can't always predict or control outcomes, but we can choose to honor and embrace the path that unfolds before us. It is my hope that you will carry the mind-body tools you learned here with you into your future and that they will bring you strength, understanding, peace, and joy wherever life takes you.

Resources

Helpful Websites

Fertility

barbarablitzer.com

Fertility and mind-body coaching; counseling. Teleconferences and Skype sessions.

infertilityworkbook.com

Downloads, information, and programs to support your infertility workbook practice.

Resolve: The National Infertility Association

resolve.org

A well-respected volunteer organization dedicated to providing information and support for individuals and couples struggling with infertility. Includes national, online, and local resources.

American Fertility Association
theafa.org
Offers a wealth of information and resources for the fertility community online.

The Society for Assisted Reproductive Technologies
sart.org
SART is an affiliate of the American Society for Reproductive Medicine. Its mission is to set standards for assisted reproductive technology. It provides statistics on IVF success rates.

American Society for Reproductive Medicine
asrm.org
ASRM is a multidisciplinary organization providing information and support for professionals and the general public. It provides patient-information sheets on a variety of topics. You can find information on the medical and psychological aspects of fertility here.

The InterNational Council on Infertility Information Dissemination, Inc.
inciid.org
A nonprofit organization that provides fertility-related information and support. Offers a newsletter, online chats, and articles about emotional, physical, and practical issues.

Centers for Disease Control and Prevention
cdc.gov/art/
A source for statistics on the success rates of infertility clinics.

The American Congress of Obstetricians and Gynecologists
www.acog.org
ACOG provides patient information on lifestyle management for women trying to conceive and for pregnant women. Publications on preconception health include information on food choice and weight.

Adoption

American Academy of Adoption Attorneys
adoptionattorneys.org
Lists attorneys with expertise in adoption and provides guidance in the legal matters to be considered when pursuing adoption. Provides a directory of adoption agencies.

www.adoption.com
Addresses many adoption-related issues. Links to additional resources and information.

General Mental Health

Anxiety Disorder Association of America
www.adaa.org
A nonprofit dedicated to preventing and treating anxiety disorders.

National Association of Cognitive-Behavioral Therapists
nacbt.org
Materials, information, and support related to cognitive behavioral therapy.

National Institute of Mental Health
nimh.nih.gov
Information about mental health diagnosis, research, and treatment.

Meditation, Mindfulness, and Stress Reduction

Bio-Medical Instruments, Inc.
bio-medical.com
A biofeedback supply company from which you can purchase portable biofeedback equipment to measure hand temperature. The stress thermometer to be used with autogenics can be purchased here.

Independent Meditation Center Guide
gosit.org
Information, products, and resources for all types of meditation.

Additional Reading

Radical Acceptance:Embracing Your Life with the Heart of a Buddha, by Tara Brach. New York: Bantam. 2003.

The Miracle of Mindfulness, by Thich Nhat Hanh. Boston: Beacon. 1999.

Arriving at Your Own Door: 108 Lessons in Mindfulness, by Jon Kabat-Zinn. New York: Hyperion. 2007.

The Relaxation and Stress Reduction Workbook, 6th edition, by Martha Davis, Elizabeth Robbins Eshelman, and Matthew McKay. Oakland, CA: New Harbinger Publications. 2008.

The Infertility Cure, by Randine Lewis. New York: Little, Brown and Company. 2004.

100 Questions and Answers about Infertility, by John D. Gordon and Michael DiMattina. Sudbury, MA: Jones and Bartlett Publishers. 2008.

The Infertility Survival Handbook, by Elizabeth Swire Falker. New York: Riverhead Books. 2004.

References

Al-Hasani, S., and Khaled Zohni. 2008. The overlooked role of obesity in infertility. *Journal of Family and Reproductive Health* 2 (3): 115–122.

American Psychiatric Association. 2000. *Diagnostic and Statistical Manual of Mental Disorders*. 4th ed. Text rev. Washington, DC: American Psychiatric Association.

Barbieri, R. L. 2001. The initial fertility consultation: Recommendations concerning cigarette smoking, body mass index, and alcohol and caffeine consumption. *American Journal of Obstetrics and Gynecology* 185 (5): 1168–73.

Barbieri, R. L., A. D. Domar, and K. R. Loughlin. 2000. *Six Steps to Increased Fertility: An Integrated Medical and Mind/Body Program to Promote Conception*. New York: Simon and Schuster.

Begley, S. 2007. *Train Your Mind, Change Your Brain*. New York: Ballantine.

Benson, H. 1983. The relaxation response: Its subjective and objective historical precedents and physiology. *Trends in Neurosciences* 6: 281–84.

Benson, H., and W. Proctor. 2010. *Relaxation Revolution.* Scribner: New York.

Borkovec, T. D., and E. Costello. 1993. Efficacy of applied relaxation and cognitive-behavioral therapy in the treatment of generalized anxiety disorder. *Journal of Consulting and Clinical Psychology* 61 (4): 611–19.

Buck Louis, G. M., K. J. Lum, R. Sundaram, Z. Chen, S. Kim, C. D. Lynch, E. F. Schisterman, and C. Pyper. 2011. Stress reduces conception probabilities across the fertile window: Evidence in support of relaxation. *Fertility and Sterility* 95 (7): 2184–9.

Centers for Disease Control and Prevention 2011. Infertility FAQs. Accessed April 26. http://www.cdc.gov/reproductivehealth/Infertility/index.htm#3.

Dechanet, C., T. Anahory, J. C. Mathieu Daude, X. Quantin, L. Reyftmann, S. Hamamah, B. Hedon, and H. Dechaud. 2011. Effects of cigarette smoking on reproduction. *Human Reproduction Update* 17 (1): 76–95.

DeRubeis, R. J., and P. Crits-Christoph. 1998. Empirically supported individual and group psychological treatments for adult mental disorders. *Journal of Consulting and Clinical Psychology* 66: 37–52.

Dobson, K. S. 1989. A meta-analysis of the efficacy of cognitive therapy for depression. *Journal of Consulting and Clinical Psychology* 57 (3): 414–19.

Domar, A. 2002. *Conquering Infertility.* New York: Viking.

Domar, A., D. Clapp, E. Slawsby, J. Dusek, B. Kessel, and M. Freizinger. 2000. Impact of group psychological interventions on pregnancy rates in infertile women. *Fertility and Sterility* 73 (4): 805–11.

Domar, A., and J. Nikolovski. 2009. Study showing link between stress and increased infertility, presented at the American Society for Reproductive Medicine's 65th Annual Meeting, Atlanta, October 19.

Durham, R. C., J. A. Chambers, R. R. MacDonald, K. G. Power, and K. Major. 2003. Does cognitive-behavioral therapy influence the long-term outcome of generalized anxiety disorder? An 8–14-year follow-up of two clinical trials. *Psychological Medicine* 33: 499–509.

Ebbesen, S. M. S., R. Zachariae, M. Y. Mehlsen, D. Thomsen, A. Hoejgaard, L. Ottosen, T. Petersen, and H. J. Ingerslev. 2009. Stressful life events are associated with a poor in-vitro fertilization (IVF) outcome: A prospective study. *Human Reproduction* 24 (9): 2173–82.

Fedorcsák, P., P. O. Dale, R. Storeng, G. Ertzeid, S. Bjercke, N. Oldereid, A. K. Omland, T. Abyholm, and T. Tanbo. 2004. Impact of overweight and underweight on assisted reproduction treatment. *Human Reproduction* 19 (11): 2523–28.

Gendlin, E. T. 1981. *Focusing.* Rev. ed. New York: Bantam Dell.

Gottman, J., and N. Silver. 2000. *The Seven Principles for Making Marriage Work.* New York: Three Rivers Press.

Gould, R. A., M. W. Otto, M. H. Pollack, and L. Yap. 1997. Cognitive behavioral and pharmacological treatment of generalized anxiety disorder: A preliminary meta-analysis. *Behavior Therapy* 28 (2): 285–305.

Hakim, R. B., R. H. Gray, and H. Zacur. 1998. Alcohol and caffeine consumption and decreased fertility. *Fertility and Sterility* 70 (4): 632–37.

Hallowell, E. M. 1998. *Worry*. New York: Ballantine.

Hollon, S. D., R. J. DeRubeis, R. C. Shelton, J. D. Amsterdam, R. M. Salomon, J. P. O'Reardon, M. L. Lovett, P. R. Young, K. L. Haman, B. B. Freeman, and R. Gallop. 2005. Prevention of relapse following cognitive therapy vs. medications in moderate to severe depression. *Archives of General Psychology* 62: 417–22.

Kabat-Zinn, J. A., A. O. Massion, J. Kristeller, L. G. Peterson, K. E. Fletcher, L. Pbert, W. R. Lenderking, and S. F. Santorelli. 1992. Effectiveness of a meditation-based stress reduction program in the treatment of anxiety disorders. *American Journal of Psychiatry* 149: 936–43.

Luke, B., M. B. Brown, J. E. Stern, S. A. Missmer, V. Y. Fujimoto, R. Leach, and SART Writing Group. 2011. Female obesity adversely affects assisted reproductive technology (ART) pregnancy and live birth rates. *Human Reproduction* 26 (1): 245–52.

Manheimer, E., G. Zhang, L. Udoff, A. Haramati, P. Langenberg, B. M. Berman, and L. M. Bouter. 2008. Effects of acupuncture on rates of pregnancy and live birth among women undergoing in vitro fertilisation: Systematic review and meta-analysis. *British Medical Journal* 336 (7643): 545-49.

Nhat Hanh, Thich. 1993. *The Blooming of a Lotus: Guided Meditation for Achieving the Miracle of Mindfulness*. Translated by Annabel Laity. Boston: Beacon Press.

Pennebaker, J. W. 2002. "Writing, Social Processes, and Psychotherapy: From Past to Future." In *The Writing Cure: How Expressive Writing Promotes Health and Emotional Well-Being*, edited by Stephen J. Lepore and Joshua M. Smyth. Washington, DC: American Psychological Association.

Pennebaker, J. W., J. K. Kiecolt-Glaser, and R. Glaser. 1988. Disclosure of traumas and immune function: Health implications for psychotherapy. *Journal of Consulting and Clinical Psychology* 56 (2): 239–45.

Roizen, M. 2011. Personal communication via e-mail, July 1.

Seigel, D. J. 2010. *Mindsight*. New York: Bantam.

Sendak, M. 1963. *Where the Wild Things Are*. New York: Harper and Row.

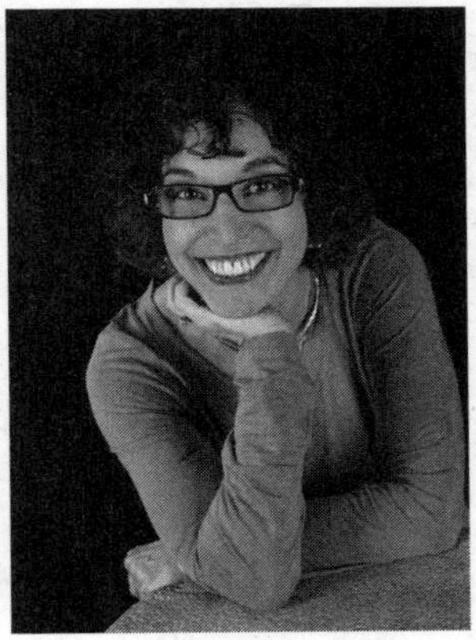

Barbara Blitzer, LCSW-C, MEd, is a licensed clinical social worker and psychotherapist who pioneered the integration of mind-body approaches with psychotherapy to reduce stress and enhance fertility. She has worked with RESOLVE: The National Infertility Association, fertility clinics, and in her own private practice in the Washington, DC, area. She is a professional member of the American Society for Reproductive Medicine, RESOLVE, The National Association of Social Workers, and The Greater Washington Clinical Society. Her work has been cited in the *Washington Post, Washington Woman,* and in other media outlets. Visit her online at www.barbarablitzer.com.

Foreword writer **Rafat A. Abbasi, MD, FACOG,** is board-certified in obstetrics and gynecology, as well as in reproductive endocrinology and infertility. She is a reproductive endocrinology physician at Columbia Fertility Associates and chair of the department of gynecology at Suburban Hospital in Bethesda, MD.